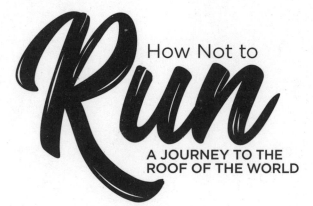

How Not to

Run

A JOURNEY TO THE
ROOF OF THE WORLD

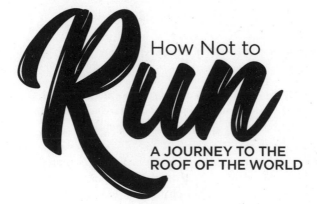

How Not to
Run

A JOURNEY TO THE
ROOF OF THE WORLD

SHAUNEY WATSON

First published by Pitch Publishing, 2018

Pitch Publishing
A2 Yeoman Gate
Yeoman Way
Worthing
Sussex
BN13 3QZ
www.pitchpublishing.co.uk
info@pitchpublishing.co.uk

A CIP catalogue record is available for this book
from the British Library.

ISBN 978-1-78531-453-7

Typesetting and origination by Pitch Publishing
Printed and bound in India by Replika Press Pvt. Ltd.

Contents

It wasn't supposed to be like this

It's 5pm Nepalese time and I can barely breathe for vomiting so hard. I'm doubled over a hole in the floor of a cold, stone room, heaving as if my internal organs are intent on leaving my body.

It wouldn't be so bad if I was in a clean bathroom that didn't have a floor covered in pee, or if I was throwing up into a toilet that wasn't a hole in the ground used by the many travellers who had passed through that day. It wouldn't even have been as bad if the temperature wasn't a ridiculous -17°C or if I wasn't 5,164 metres above sea level.

A lot of things could have been better at 5pm this fine, cold evening at the old Everest Base Camp. But one thing which definitely made everything worse was the small, inconvenient fact that I had a full 26.2-mile marathon to tackle the next morning and an entire night of food poisoning-related sickness and diarrhoea in front of me.

It was never supposed to be like this, and it almost wasn't.

Chapter One

Alcohol and the internet

November 2017

There was another rum and Coke in my hand. I definitely hadn't ordered one, I was sure.

I looked at the barman with a quizzical expression and he laughed while flicking a bottle up over his arm to make someone's cocktail. With a shrug I settled myself on the bar stool in the corner. I had a feeling I was going to be here a while and I can't say I was particularly perturbed by this turn of events. Hitching my hiking boots on the bar stool footrest with a contented sigh, I watched the folk around the bar – many of whom I could now consider real friends – and smiled ruefully at their raucous celebrations.

The Nepalese barman laughing and joking with customers on the opposite side of the bar to me was quite possibly the coolest barman I had ever met. In fact, it's unlikely I will come across a cooler barman. He ducked under the bar to take his shot on the pool table and I shifted to let him past.

Our vivacious group were currently making merry in what is apparently the highest Irish pub in the world. The walls of this little pub are covered in flags and memorabilia from the many, many trekkers who had passed through its doors. The flags had likely seen many a party like the one going on tonight. Later in the evening the electricity would cut out, which is a regular occurrence in Namche Bazaar, and the barman would play his guitar and sing to us. But for now, being the girl sitting at the end of the bar, contentedly looking on, I was handed a phone full of music and a set of speakers and was told to keep everyone dancing.

I was surprised to have yet another rum and Coke plonked down in front of me ten minutes later, by a drunk but very kind man from my group. Really, I had tried to stress during this trip that, though I may like rum and Coke, it regularly led to reckless decision-making on my part. In hindsight, I thought, as I sipped it, my reckless decision-making isn't like everyone else's. I'm not talking, 'Let's steal this traffic cone and take it home' at 3am after a heavy Friday night.

It's far more: 'Let's wholeheartedly decide to do something physically and outrageously demanding, and design it in such a way I can't allow myself to back out. Because that sounds like it won't drive me to self-induced misery and near insanity at all.' Then again, I smiled to myself, if it weren't for a couple of glasses of rum and Coke, the last four crazy, painful, awe-inspiring and incredible weeks would never have happened to me. Perhaps Captain Morgan deserves a little bit of recognition for that one.

Two years previously

There I was, a whole two years ago, also sitting with a rum and Coke in my hand, on one of the sofas in my mum and dad's house. Google was open on the laptop in front of me and, as had so often been the case over the last few weeks, I was feeling particularly uneasy with myself.

I was 19 going on 20 and at that tricky point where you're wondering what the hell you're doing with your life. Part of you is trying to convince yourself you've got your shit together, while the other part considers surviving on a family-sized pack of Walkers crisps and watching Jeremy Kyle reruns all day might be easier than adult life. Or at least the semi-adult life I appeared to be attempting to lead.

Being an over-thinking, control-freak stress-head with no social skills and limited finances (gentlemen, form an orderly queue please), I had taken up running about 18 months earlier. It gave me something I could structure and control and, best of all, I didn't have to speak to anyone while I did it.

I say I 'took up' running but that's bullshit. I had been a keen horse rider my whole life and liked to keep fit so I could at least stay in the saddle more than I hit the ground. For this reason I decided to go for a light one-mile jog one day, got hopelessly lost and ended up doing six miles. This is testimony to my excellent navigational skills and quite possibly why I really should have known better than to consider fell running 18 months later. You know, running in those places where you need a map and compass and things.

Anyway, managing to run six miles startled me, and it got me thinking. Perhaps I could do a ten-kilometre race; wouldn't that be exciting! Of course, I got curious and entered one, and once I successfully completed it I got that rush of excitement where you begin to wonder what else you can manage. A half-marathon, perhaps? Like most newbie runners, the excitement of managing something new and physically demanding kept me setting new challenges for myself and so, once the half was accomplished, I inevitably ended up deciding to tackle a marathon for charity.

It's worth back-tracking a year or two here to explain.

Studying various psychological therapies after high school, I had come to learn a little about post-traumatic stress disorder (PTSD), the psychological condition which can affect anyone who has suffered a trauma. For those it affects, the memory of the event isn't collected and stored in a functionable way in the brain. Instead, the memory 'shatters', with fragments of it lodging in areas of the mind in which they cannot be accepted. This leads to debilitating symptoms such as flashbacks, whereby the event is essentially lived all over again, not to mention the behaviour change and relationship breakdowns that can and usually do happen as well.

I have no mental illness to speak of but just knowing what goes on in my own head, from being a nervous child, depressingly moody teenager and now a stressy young adult, I know how difficult it is to work with a temperamental mind. And that's just with normal, day-to-day things! I can only imagine the hell of having PTSD.

It wasn't long before I found out what a growing problem PTSD was in soldiers, how little support was in place for ex-soldiers and how bad this problem was likely to become in the future.

While the US collects data on soldiers suffering mental illness after they have left the military system, the UK's Ministry of Defence (MOD) doesn't. This means the UK's statistics on soldiers suffering from PTSD come from data collected on soldiers still under the care of the MOD and not from veterans in the years after retirement.

The MOD's statistics show that from 2015 to 2016, 0.18 per cent of the armed forces had an initial assessment for PTSD, and from 2016 to 2017 this rose to 0.19 per cent. But PTSD can either lie dormant or simply unrecognised in a person for five-plus years before it surfaces or the person finally seeks help. When you take this into account, it becomes clear that the MOD's statistics on mental illness among veterans are likely to be way off the mark.

Keystone US studies have found PTSD affects up to 18 per cent of combat veterans, and when you consider the unique factors involved in warfare these days, this statistic is unsurprising. From the fear of sustained attack, biological and chemical weapons and uncovering human remains, to having a friend and colleague shot or injured in front of you or being shot or injured yourself, the list of those factors is extensive. Furthermore, deployment length is often unknown and multiple deployments are always likely.

A study by the King's Centre for Military Health Research of 4,928 UK armed forces personnel deployed in Iraq in 2003 found that 12 per cent admitted to being violent after returning home. Often this was triggered by flashbacks of combat and trauma.

Once soldiers have retired from the armed forces, they are left with the daunting task of trying to establish a functioning civilian life. This can be a struggle even for those veterans not challenged by physical or mental illness, but for those suffering from acute stress or PTSD, the task can be overwhelming.

Combat Stress is a veterans' mental health charity dedicated to helping soldiers and veterans suffering with mental illness. The demand for its services has grown massively in the last few years due to the increase in the number of veterans from recent conflicts beginning to seek the charity's help.

A better awareness and understanding of mental illness in soldiers has helped to increase the number of veterans seeking help, but the stigma still remains at military unit level. The charity estimates that referrals will continue to rise over the next ten years as it deals with the aftermath of Iraq and Afghanistan.

Through therapeutic work, complete remission can be achieved in 30–50 per cent of cases, and partial improvement can be expected in most.

Though it is often said that prevention is better than cure, it's difficult to see how to prevent PTSD occurring in soldiers facing such volatile environments. Training programmes have been developed to try to prepare soldiers for combat and other stress factors related to deployment, and to reduce their risk of exposure to traumatic events, e.g. military sexual trauma. Part of each programme trains service personnel how to respond to such events should they occur.

The next step from here is trying to detect and treat mental disorders in the early stages. Acute Stress Disorder often presents before the onset of chronic PTSD. It has been found that intervening at this stage can significantly reduce symptoms and prevent PTSD taking hold.

Interventions can be implemented immediately after trauma and this has also been shown to reduce the risk of PTSD developing.

Of course, this all relies on symptoms being detected instantly and acted upon quickly which often isn't the case, sadly.

Though we may not be at war at the moment, the effects of conflicts over the last 20 to 50 years are still being felt across the veteran community. Ex-soldiers without the support they need so often reach the point at which they feel they can't keep going. It's all too common to hear of another soldier having taken his or her own life.

I find this more than just sad, more than just unfair; I find it bloody despicable. These men and women join our military to serve our country because they feel it's right or honourable or their duty, and they come out of it with these mental scars which prevent them from moving on into normal civilian life, prevent them from enjoying being with their families, prevent them from living. And the system they work for does so little to help or support them in the years after service. PTSD isn't a new thing – we've known about it since the Great War – so why isn't more being done?

This played on my mind for a long time after studying it, and what bugged me was the fact that I couldn't really do anything about it. I wasn't likely to be in any kind of government position where I could try to make a change. Nor was I likely to be involved in any kind of mental health care regime designed for recovering PTSD sufferers.

All I could do that *might* help was run. Maybe, through this, I could at least raise money for other people in the right sectors who could then do something about it. I decided that the charity I had heard of most while studying PTSD was Combat Stress, and I signed up for the Loch Ness Marathon to raise some money for them. As any marathon runner knows, when you sign up for that first marathon there is some serious doubt that runs through your mind (and body) because a marathon is the biggest thing a human body can physically do, isn't it? Of course it's not, and any marathon runner will tell you how perfectly achievable it is ... if you put the work in.

But then BANG! The weeks of training and all the hype around the marathon are over, and you're dropped from a great height back down to earth. It was such a big deal for me for about five months, raising money while training and training and training, and then ... nothing. And this crash landing back down to earth, I would later find out, is the 'post-marathon blues stage' of the whole marathon experience. Everyone will fail to warn you about this stage, trust me.

And so here you are, all caught up. Maybe you can better understand the feelings I was having as I sat here on mum and dad's sofa, in front of a laptop with a glass full of rum and Coke, a heart full of post-mara blues, and a head full of lifestyle choices featuring Jeremy Kyle reruns.

I was frustrated, too. The marathon had raised £750 for Combat Stress, which was great. I was extremely humbled by people's generosity. But in the great scheme of things, that wasn't going to do very much. Surely there was more I could do?

I can't quite recall how I found HorseBack UK. I would have read about it somewhere, I'm sure. What I do recall is the idea of this little charity sticking in my mind and refusing to leave.

The work Combat Stress does is life-altering as well as life-saving, and it is a charity I feel deserves as much recognition as possible. And this is something its board and thousands of staff work hard towards. But I decided if I was to carry on fundraising for this cause I wanted to find a charity small enough to go and see the inner workings, see precisely where the money raised goes, speak to the owners and hear the passion from the creators and benefactors themselves.

HorseBack UK was this charity. With a small team of dedicated staff in the hills of Aboyne in Scotland, HorseBack UK takes in groups of combat veterans suffering from mental or physical trauma and teaches them to work with the 30 or so horses on the 'ranch'. They learn new skills in the form of equestrianism on the farm and conservation work on the estate. From learning horsemanship to repairing fences and handling falcons, the courses at HorseBack UK aim to inspire recovery, helping veterans to regain their self-esteem while learning coping strategies, life skills and lasting resilience.

The veterans get the opportunity to regain focus and purpose, to put some distance between themselves and the world they now find themselves suffocated by and be part of the atmosphere, banter and kinship they were so used to during their military careers.

Founders Jock and Emma Hutchison registered HorseBack UK as an official charity in 2009 after initially looking to set up a trekking centre in the Highlands of Scotland. Jock, a former marine, and Emma, a former police officer, were looking to settle down to a quiet country life when they invited some friends with military backgrounds to their new home in Aboyne. It was while in front of the bonfire one night that their friends mentioned how amazing this place would be for the guys coming back from Afghanistan with physical and mental war wounds. The period 2008 to 2009 had been one of the worst for fatalities and life-changing injuries in soldiers in Afghanistan. The seed was planted.

Initially looking to the oil industry to gain some sponsorship to run their first course for Afghanistan veterans, Jock and Emma were turned down. This was when they changed tack slightly and, rather than looking for sponsorship, contacted Royal Marines 45 Commando directly to gauge interest in the idea. 45 Commando had had a devastating two-year period, losing nine comrades and having others with life-changing injuries. The Royal Marines unit jumped at the opportunity to send some of their recovering soldiers to the ranch.

HorseBack UK has grown considerably over the years since these first shaky steps. Being one of the first charities to gain funding from Help for Heroes, and now with a dedicated team of volunteers and staff around them, it has two arenas, a round pen, a converted farm steading and accommodation for the men and women attending its courses. It only takes talking to one of the guys on a course at HorseBack to know how truly worth it the time and effort to build this place up has been. The work this small charity does is so important to the men and women who pass through its doors, quite literally saving the lives of those who thought they were lost.

I wanted to be able to help. But I couldn't do another fundraising road marathon; that was a certainty. The whole point of the first one was the fact that I didn't think I could do it and therefore I assumed other people would doubt me, too. To me, that seemed worth sponsoring. I don't really see the point in sponsoring someone to do something that's a dead cert. Where's the challenge? So if I was going to try to raise more money it would have to be through something I didn't think I could do.

Cue more Captain Morgan's, Google, and a website featuring the Everest Marathon. A few minutes of reading and I decided this was the best-looking race on the whole of the internet. I had a buzzy sense of excitement beginning to grow as I read on. What did I need to have done? Only a few ultramarathons, a bit of mountain experience and some trail-racing experience: you know, all the things I'd never done in my life before. Hell, a few months ago I couldn't even go for a one-mile jog without getting lost. I was now supposed to be trusted on a mountain on my own!

But yes! This race sounded brilliantly mental. The race itself involved two weeks of trekking to the start line with temperatures ranging from -20°C to +30°C in the space of a day, and then an entire marathon with half the oxygen your body needs, over terrain to make your ankles cry.

In the space of 15 minutes I had decided I was doing it. The next race was 2017 which gave me two years to do all those ridiculous things they wanted on my CV. Plenty of time!

Being the least patient person I know, the next website I visited was the Scottish Running Guide, on the hunt for my first ultramarathon. Might as well start as I meant to go on!

I soon found one ... and entered it about ten minutes later. It was all so wonderfully exciting!

Now, let's all just bear in mind at this point I had done *one* road marathon. That's 26.2 miles of smooth, even surface over a few undulating hills. Therefore, my decision to enter a 55-mile race (yes, 55 miles) in just five months' time was probably foolhardy at best. Planning to do the Everest Marathon in 24 months' time was even more so. But Google and my good old Captain Morgan's said it was a good idea, and, that evening, that was good enough for me ... hiccup ...

Chapter Two

Skinny dipping by moonlight

January 2016

'What is wrong with you?' I groaned to myself at 2am this cold January morning while pulling on one filthy trainer. 'Normal people don't do this. They really, really, really ... eugh why's it so cohhhhhhld ... really, really don't.' Lace tightened, next trainer on. I didn't want to do this. Like, I *really* didn't want to do this. It was cold, dark and wet outside and I had only just woken up. My body was screaming at me to go back to bed and that was before I even considered the 18 miles I had stretching out in front of me.

Even using my phone to play annoyingly motivational music as my alarm, set to vibrate and placed on the radiator at the opposite side of my bedroom, wasn't enough to rouse me from the zombified state I currently found myself in.

Head down, dragging my feet, I slumped out into the pitch dark, still grumbling and cursing to myself as I made my way up the wooded track to the main road. My head torch was doing a shockingly bad job of lighting the riveted track in front of me which I figured meant it needed new batteries. Again, why was I doing this? The ditches at either side of the track were brimming with black, glassy water, much like almost every ditch in the country, I expected. We had had a month of severe rain with almost every part of Scotland flooding. Huge areas of land had disappeared under more rainwater than I'd seen in my life. But it had stopped raining a week previously and most of the water was draining away now. Or, for the sake of this morning's run, I hoped it had.

It took a good three miles before my mental grumbling subsided and I settled into an okay-ish rhythm. It was 2.30am and -5°C. I wasn't bouncing. However, I wasn't falling apart either. The soggy fields and trees were all dimly lit by moonlight, sparkling in the cold, and there were no cars on the road so I didn't need my head torch switched on the whole time at least. These were the sorts of little things that made an early morning long run before work at 9am bearable.

However, seven miles came around and my shins were starting to twinge. You know that itchy way just-healing shin splints get just before they bugger up again? I had only been introduced to this feeling in the last two or three months so I still wasn't sensible enough to ease up when I felt it. Pounding down the tarmac towards a road which had been shut a week ago due to flooding, I tried really hard to ignore the shooting pain starting to creep up the inside of one of my shins from my ankle. But, despite my best efforts, it was all I was really thinking about. In hindsight, it might have been worth taking a look around at my dimly moonlit surroundings for a second instead.

That road, I thought, couldn't possibly still be flooded. Think again, Shauney. I started down it for a short distance before my trainers started splashing in about two inches of water. That was okay, though. It was too cold to feel my feet anyway so what did wet socks matter? The two inches, however, quickly grew to ankle depth which was less than satisfactory. I reasoned with myself: if this is as deep as it gets, I can deal with that. It was only eight miles to home now, I was sure I had dealt with worse.

By the time the freezing-cold water was creeping up my calves I realised I'd made a big mistake in not checking that all the roads were no longer flooded before setting out on this foolhardy, long run. But if I turned around now, I would either have to head back the way I'd come which was longer than the distance I had left to go, or I could head further up the main road to go the long way round, again adding unnecessary miles. My other option: I could hope that this was as deep as the water got and plough on regardless.

Of course, of those options I picked the most stubborn and idiotic and no, as a point of interest, that wasn't as deep as the water got. By the time I was wading through waist high, freezing-cold water I wasn't just questioning my sanity but also whether my legs would ever recover, given the fact that they now felt sort of hollow and echoey. There were vibrations going through them with every slow footstep as if my legs were planks of wood.

'You're an idiot. A total bloody idiot. WHY would that seem like a good idea?' I shivered to myself as I finally waded out the other side a half-mile later. I don't think I stopped cursing myself all the way home. With water squelching from my trainers with every step, I was glad of the numbness currently enfolding my feet. The blisters would have been impressively painful otherwise!

My dad was getting ready for work when I eventually trundled back down the track, still soggy and shivering having taken a lot longer than normal to run the last eight miles after my half-mile wading exercise. He sighed, shaking his head and muttering something about wondering where he and mum had found me.

Icing the joints is good for them, I reasoned. My shin splints weren't bothering me after it, anyway! I chalked it up to a successful learning curve as I attempted to warm my frozen butt on the stove. The fact that most of my toes didn't return to normal functioning ability for a few days was, of course, by the by, as was the fact that the 18 miles had taken me almost four hours. I was resolutely determined not to admit that my complete lack of common sense was a bad thing. I totally had this training thing down. As long as I didn't remind myself of the fact Glasgow to Edinburgh was now just two months away and my legs seemed to be injured more than they were fixed, I could convince myself I was doing okay.

February 2016

Praise all things wonderful! 23 miles on Sunday and it went smooth as a baby's bum — hallelujah!, it went amazingly. Not so much as a twinge anywhere. Sure, my knee was sore later and my shin a bit iffy, but that was later not during the run! It took more out of me than I thought though. I loosened things off in the gym last night and came away feeling shaky and a bit sick. All day I hadn't been able to muster up all that much energy so by the time I was finished in the gym I could barely keep my eyes open.

I've now come up with a plan for the rest of my training weeks. I found a blog by an ultrarunner who basically said if you have trained for a marathon you can bounce straight into a 50-mile ultra. He did with just three weeks' training to prepare. As long as you can do two 20-mile runs back to back and a single 30-mile run you're good for a 50-mile race. It won't look pretty, but you'll get through it! And this news was good enough for me!

It amazes me, reading this now as I put together this chapter, to see how utterly foolhardy I was about my body, and what I would put it through. I fully expected it to perform better every time I ran, to be stronger every time I exercised and be generally more streamlined every time I trained. With no heed for rest or recuperation, I adopted a mindset somewhere between obsession and sadism. I was genuinely angry at my body whenever it failed me and only ever happy when, by some miracle, I seemed to have improved.

March 2016

I had planned to do five runs throughout the second week of Feb, before giving myself the first few days of the third week to rest. I would then tackle the first of these big runs. I got through the five runs I had planned but only just. I was coming down with some bug on the Saturday and just scraped through Sunday's run before the flu hit me like a bloody wrecking ball. I was ill to the point I couldn't ride my horses or go to work, which is unheard of! It pushed training back a full week and was still lingering at the beginning of last week. But, as Sunday was the 28th and I had till the 1st of March to pull out of this damned ultra, I would do the two back-to-back 20-mile runs on Friday and Saturday and that would be the true test. If I could get through essentially 40 miles of the 55 I would have to do in April then it was on. But I HAD to be able to do them both in full with no injuries.

Well, it's now the 1st of March and I'm more than delighted to say: holy shit I did it! Surprised the hell out of myself when I was still alive on Sunday. It had been a 4.30am start on the Friday to ride and do yard duties, work 9am till 5pm (during which time I became increasingly nervous). Then, setting off at 6pm, I did my first 20 miles in just under four hours. The next morning I did my yard duties quickly, didn't even ride, and set off at 9am. I had company for the last seven miles but, Christ, it was tough! Mainly because my body just seemed to be refusing of its own accord. The last two miles, however, I dug deep and did them at a pace I would never have expected from myself at the end of 40 miles. My last was an eight--minute mile! That was pure stubbornness and stroppiness at feeling so crap if I'm honest!

And then, being 20 and not very wise, I went on a night out, hitting the clubs and not getting back till 4am ...

Sunday was a tired blur but I thought just doing some weights in the gym would have me back to normal. Will I ever learn?! The gym was another shaky, weak experience leaving me feeling sick again. But on the bright side — the race is on!

The entire five months of training for Glasgow to Edinburgh was a rollercoaster of, 'Yay, I did it!' to, 'Jesus Christ, why am I falling apart again?' Five days after that blog entry I was kicked in the leg by a horse and foolishly pushed through an 18-mile run the next day. By the time I finished, the leg would hardly bear any weight. But with the same hare-brained defiance I had held on to throughout my training, I set out on, and finished, the 30-mile run the following weekend after a stressful week of making my leg better. Well, almost, anyway. I was only slightly leaning on the ibuprofen, paracetamol, ibu-gel and tape.

Somehow – and God knows how when you look at what I put my poor body through – 1 April rolled around and I was still resolutely entered in the race.

April 2016

Well, here I am, sitting at work, about to close up, wondering what tomorrow will hold. I get on a train in an hour and a half for Glasgow, I start my run in 16 hours and hopefully finish it 27 hours from now. This is a bit of a rushed diary entry as I'm about to get picked up straight after closing up tonight, but I am wondering what the hell I've done ... still.

Chapter Three

Young, blonde and teary-eyed will get you a long way

It would be fair to say my upbringing had been, not sheltered, but definitely quiet. I was a country girl to the core and even joining a bigger gym in my nearest city and going out for the odd run while there showed I was less street-savvy chic and more babe in the Big City. Heavy traffic scared the bejesus out of me. Give me a barbed wire fence and a fast-flowing river to cross any day. I had that shit down by the age of ten.

Perhaps, in hindsight, setting out to get to Glasgow on my own the night before my first ultramarathon was not the wisest of moves. If heavy traffic scared me, it was nothing compared to the thought of navigating three train stations. And yet, here I was, at Edinburgh train station, frantically pacing between the barriers, trying to decide which bloody one I was supposed to go through. Ticket, screen, train, ticket, screen, train – it didn't matter how many times I checked each, nothing seemed to match.

'How have I managed to get to 20 years of age without knowing how to get on a bloody train?' I hissed to myself through clenched teeth as I tried to keep my stomach in place.

With what I thought was only five minutes till my train was due to leave, I picked the train that sounded like the best match and tried my best to carry my bags as though I totally knew what I was doing. Before I boarded, I spotted a hi-vis tabard-wearing man strolling up the platform. Ah, the comfort of an authoritative figure in such surroundings! I asked him if this train I was so confidently about to board was going to Glasgow Charing Cross.

'No, love,' he said, seemingly bored with my inadequately challenging question. 'That one just left a couple of minutes ago. This one's going to Glasgow Queen Street.'

Ah, fuck.

The last call was being shouted for Glasgow Queen Street. The hi-vis man was wandering off.

'Fuck, fuck, fuckety fuck.' In a panic, I boarded and sat down on the first available seat. What was I doing? I looked out of the window into the darkness as the train began to move, and watched as the brick walls began to pass. I had no idea how far Queen Street was from Charing Cross, or how far it was from my hostel for that matter!

The window was black now with only streams of rain running across the glass.

Did I even know where my hostel was? And that was if I even got to Glasgow and wasn't chucked off the train for not having the right ticket. At that thought, I promptly burst into tears. This whole thing was a stupid idea. I was on the wrong train, in the middle of Scotland, completely on my own, with no money. Like, seriously, the phrase 'strapped for cash' didn't even begin to describe my financial situation at that point. And if I ended up in the right place, I was to run 55 miles tomorrow on a crushed foot (to be explained) and kicked-in thigh. What was I thinking?

A man sat down in the seat opposite me, unaware until the last second I was trying to quietly have an emotional breakdown, mascara undoubtedly running eye to chin by now.

Out of the corner of my eye I could see his slightly panic-stricken face, unsure of whether to awkwardly get up again and find another seat or try to pretend he hadn't noticed and stay put. He decided on the latter.

'Tickets, please,' the bored tone of the ticket inspector carried up the train a few minutes later. Oh God, this was awful. Could I hide? No, he'd seen me. Shit.

Thankfully, and by some miracle, the slightly panic-stricken man opposite me had lost his ticket and in the ensuing problem-solving conversation between him and the bored ticket inspector, I was overlooked. I know, right! When does that ever happen?

Still sniffling, I did my best to blend into the seat for the rest of the ride and not think about the fact I had to run this entire train journey tomorrow. I mean, really, when you think about it, only a runner would consider taking a train somewhere in order to run back to where they started. It was totally idiotic.

Sitting on this train tonight, I was scared. Petrified, actually. Barely any of my six months of training had gone to plan. I had scraped through with what I felt was the bare minimum I needed for this race, though it's probably worth mentioning that I didn't have a clue what I was doing when it came to training for an ultra.

This 'bare minimum' training might have given me a glimmer of hope, though, had it not been for that horse kick I'd taken to the side of my thigh, putting my knee out. The bugger left a hefty hoof-shaped bruise, too! But I'd made it through the 30-miler after that so I could have convinced myself I didn't have a problem had it not been for the second horse-related incident which left my foot thoroughly trodden on just ten days before the race. I couldn't believe the timing of everything. Especially given the fact that my feet are always being trodden on and are never a problem! I was still hobbling three days later, feeling very, very sorry for myself. My list of horse- and running-related injuries had become so long and repetitive, my family were all sick to the back teeth of me.

'It started as just runners' knee, you see, but now there's shin splints, and then there was that stress reaction in my foot ...' You can see their eyes glazing over somewhere between 'knee' and 'splints' every time.

When there had still been time in my training to make a difference, I had felt frustrated at not being able to make the changes I needed to make. But time had run out now and I had resigned myself to the fact the race was going to be an unmitigated disaster. I was somewhere between finding it completely hilarious and wanting to cry my eyes out.

Sitting here, watching the darkness and rain outside the train, I felt stupid and naive. What had made me think for one moment I could do this? I'd done one marathon and foolishly signed up for a double marathon because ... what? I was training to run one of the hardest marathons in the world at Mount Everest? Get a grip, you stupid girl! I was 20. What gave me the right to think I could do this?

You can't even get on the train you're supposed to be on!

And in the way your mind is astoundingly good at, I chastised myself and told myself how much of a fraud I was for telling people I was going to do the Everest

Marathon until there were fresh tears running down my face. This was how I arrived at the wrong station in Glasgow at 10pm this Saturday night. Thankfully, I probably looked like too much of an emotional mess to bother attacking or mugging. Not that I'm saying anything about Glasgow because it has some lovely parts but ... you know. Anyway, I wandered around, looking for a legitimate taxi to hopefully take me to my hostel.

Thankfully, the kindly taxi driver who picked me up knew where the hostel was and chatted to me on the drive there. He had heard about this crazy Glasgow to Edinburgh race being held, and by the time I arrived at my destination I was feeling a bit better.

This was not, however, to continue as the hostel receptionist claimed outright that they had not received any payment from me. I would now need to pay up front, apparently.

Given my current fragile emotional state, this news was not received very well. Needless to say, my previous payment miraculously appeared on his computer screen and, a few minutes later, I found myself alone in my room for the night. I sat on the edge of the bed with a relieved and wearisome sigh. Gods, what was I doing?

I set about the familiar process of taping my knees and shins with Rocktape and pulling socks over them to keep it all in place overnight before changing. I lay awake for a long time that night. I was *almost* 100% certain of failure tomorrow, resigned to it in a hollow way that made me question why I was frittering my life away chasing stupid concepts. Yet there was a tiny, tiny piece of me that thought it might just be possible. But that wasn't a piece I could dwell on in case the eventual failure hurt even more because of it.

All I knew right now was how terribly alone I felt. And with nobody to blame but myself, I felt even worse.

Chapter Four

Learn to love the weirdos: you're one of them

They're all weirdos. It was probably a mean, judgemental thought but I couldn't help it. Around me there were long spindly individuals with endless legs; short chunky ones with broad shoulders; bandanas and beards, braids and bunches; sci-fi-looking clothing and all kinds of strange, eclectic and presumably lucky warm-ups and rituals going on. I had never seen such a motley crew. Not even at the few running races I had attended before, where I had always felt like the odd one out.

More importantly, I continued to ponder as I stared around at my fellow Glasgow to Edinburgh ultramarathon participants, they might have seemed like weirdos to me but they were weirdos with exceptionally small running packs. Like, seriously, how in the name of hell had they managed to fit the entire minimum kit list in them? My hydration pack was not small and I'd had to full-body-wrestle the thing to get it zipped shut with everything in it.

I had been nervous before I noticed this detail but, as I stared at one man's avocado-sized backpack, I now almost needed a paper bag to breathe from. My massively oversized race pack could only be a hindrance, surely? Oh God, I was so unprepared for this.

'What am I doing?' I asked myself aloud for the sixteenth time that morning. Feeling like a frumpy little penguin compared to these athletic flamingos, I tried to follow some of their warm-ups. It sounds stupid now but at that point I didn't do warm-ups! What even constituted a warm-up? All I had really learned in the months before this about preparing my legs was that I shouldn't stretch pre- or mid-run because I wouldn't have shins left by the end. Something about temporarily weakening the muscles by stretching and since you rely on a little tension to allow them to work at their optimum, stretching pre- or mid-workout or run can lead to injury. This was as far as my knowledge of warm-ups went.

I dug some paracetamol and ibuprofen out of my worryingly large hydration pack in order to keep my hands busy as the start drew closer. FYI, swallowing down paracetamol and ibuprofen as a pre-race warm-up is not advisable. I noticed, as I became less and less able to keep the blood from draining from my face, that nobody else seemed to be having this trouble with nerves.

Some were chatting while others seemed to be getting themselves in the zone with some serious game faces on show.

And so, this is how I found myself on the start line of the Glasgow to Edinburgh double marathon: feeling like a pill-popping penguin among 50 or so racing flamingos.

It's very strange to be looking back at this exact moment. I was nervous; of course I was. And I don't doubt, despite their cool exteriors, that most of my fellow participants were nervous, too. But I had put a cap on the magnitude of the task ahead of me in my head. Perhaps it was because my only experience of this 55-mile distance had so far been motorised. I suppose it would be like somebody telling you to imagine the taste of a lemon when you've never experienced one before. Other people who have tasted lemons have told you the taste is sour but until you put a lemon on your tongue, you aren't able to mentally grasp it.

At this moment, on the start line, waiting for the 9am start, it was the little details that were stressing me out. Being the genius I am, I didn't realise the shoulder straps on my hydration pack adjusted and so I was standing on the start line with my shoulders rammed back as if I was ready to enrol in the Chinese army, all the while thinking: 'I need a pee ... but the bushes don't look very convincing ... but I really need a pee ... and my shoulders hurt ...'

Approximately 30 seconds to 9am I realised there were adjustable bits on the shoulder straps (oh, the joy!) and approximately 30 seconds after 9am I was wishing to God I had peed in one of the unconvincing bushes.

I remember having that icky 'I really could just turn around and go back to my bed' feeling I usually get at the start of a long run.

'Do I really want to do this? I don't think I do, you know' going round and round until I finally got into a rhythm. That first, hesitant stage of a run has always been one of the worst parts of running for me. At least when you're sore and breathing out of your arse you've obviously put in a strong effort and can give yourself a pat on the back. And a cookie.

However, weighing up the options of where to stop and pee occupied the first four miles of the run. There's a lot to consider in the ratio of visibility to desperation to 'steepness-of-spot' to 'is-my-arse-going-to-get-jagged-by-that-lethal-looking-bush'.

Once desperation won out, I felt momentarily better before my attention turned to the fact my legs felt tired, and 'oh Jesus we're only five or six miles in'. And here started the self-talk, the bargaining, the food planning, the water planning and the distraction tactics.

By 11 or 12 miles I was feeling alright. The self-talk had become minimal and a rhythm had kicked in. I came across another participant running at a decent pace, to pass the time talking to up until the first checkpoint at 13.1 miles. On the phone to my mum, who was by her mobile at home, waiting for my calls, I realised how great it felt to be a quarter of the way through this ultra in a fairly good time. Time had passed quickly when talking to another runner.

But then I had to hang up the phone, and as I was moving away from the checkpoint it suddenly dawned on me just how alone I was and how unimaginably far I had to go, even just to the next checkpoint. I gave myself a stern talking to, though, and got on with it for the next four miles. But time wasn't passing as quickly and the distance only seemed to get longer in my head.

'It's the patch,' I told myself. 'It's that 17/18 mile mark where you go through the patch. It'll pass.' It had been something a physio had told me: the body runs out of sugars to burn for energy, since a body can only store around 20 miles' worth of glycogen, and therefore has to switch to using fat instead. This switch feels awful. So I kept telling myself it was just the bad patch, but my thoughts continued to get darker. Every now and then I'd ask a runner who happened to be walking or running at a slower pace what mileage we were at but the answer was never encouraging.

However, at about 19 miles, something quite miraculous happened. I came across a runner who was walking and, as I passed, I slowed my pace and asked how far it was to the next checkpoint. He must have misunderstood me as he started a steady pace alongside me and thanked me for getting him back running again. We struck up a conversation as we ran. We talked about the fact he had completed a 100km race just six days before (it's incredible just how insane some of these ultrarunners are), why we were running this race, the charity I was doing it for and, importantly, Everest.

Together, we got to checkpoint two.

I was feeling more cheered by this but knew not to be too elated. It was going to be hard enough starting again after this checkpoint, knowing I had to do 33 more miles, most likely alone, and that my longest run had only been 31 miles. On the phone to mum again, she told me of the donations that had been coming in which helped to rally me on, and my chicken, mango and Lucozade Sport seemed to be sitting better than anything else during the run so far. This was also a boost.

However, starting off again was difficult. Especially given the fact it was on a slight hill at the Falkirk Wheel, a lift taking boats from one canal to another. Within 60 seconds I was, once again, trying to shut out the crappy, doom-filled brain chatter. I bargained with myself: 15 minutes of running then I could walk for two, and just keep going like that. But now even the 15-minute mark wasn't coming around fast enough, and everything just felt dire. Then, up ahead, I·spotted the red bandana and green and black T-shirt of the man I'd been running with from 19 to 22 miles. Being my usual socially awkward self I thought, 'Oh, great, I'm gaining on him but not fast enough to overtake, and if I linger, it's like "Oh, hi again" and then what? Neither he nor I will want to be stuck with another runner. Especially one we don't know!' But I wasn't about to slow my pace – I'd be lucky to make the cut-offs as it was.

So I had to suck it up and deal with the consequences later. I bet my guardian angels were crying, 'Hallelujah! She's taken the hint!' For the next 31 miles, this runner and I kept each other going at a not-too-shabby pace as well as learning almost everything about one another. We shared stories, inspiration and the pain of the run.

As we neared Edinburgh, we enjoyed some spectacular views, especially as the canal we were following passed over deep, leafy valleys. And then, in a moment I will never forget, we came to a bridge passing over a dual carriageway. There were street lights and cars and a sign pointing to 'City Centre'. It hit me. We had *run* from Glasgow and now we were in Edinburgh. I felt pure joy for the first time in a long time. Tears prickled in my eyes as I took a deep breath and the full sight dawned on me.

After this, we had just the final few miles to go. But by this point I was whole-body-weary and my mind was exhausted from the mental battle of keeping going. I was tired. Really tired.

The final few miles seemed to go on forever, longer than the whole run put together, I thought. Where was that finish line?

My running partner and now firm friend said we should walk at parts to enjoy the moment, the bubble that was this race was about to burst and this part of it should be savoured. I thought I knew what he meant but it wasn't until a good few days after the race that I really knew.

I crossed the line after 11.5 hours. It certainly wasn't fast but I had taken myself from Glasgow all the way to Edinburgh under my own steam and now had a little bit of faith I might actually manage some of the crazy things I was planning in the coming years. That was an incredible feeling.

This race was my first real taste of the 'bubble'. It wasn't hype and excitement around you, and it wasn't being carried away by an atmosphere. It was purely that state you find yourself in when pushing your body to its limit and holding it there, suspended in physical, mental, chemical and emotional toil. A beautiful pain. I guess I realised then that I *was* one of those weirdos on the start line, and always would be. And let me tell you, there's nothing wrong with being a weirdo.

Chapter Five

Don't read maps; they make you sad

Three months later

My first taste of running on rough terrain came during a race in the summer of 2016. Having shocked myself by completing the Glasgow to Edinburgh in the April, I was beginning to think that maybe, just maybe, the Everest Marathon might be achievable. And by this I mean it wasn't now galaxies away – just the distance of a few planets.

So, consulting the faintly ridiculous list of requirements with a new sense of vigour, I decided off-road was the way to go and entered the Lairig Ghru Ultra. It was an ultramarathon only by a mile or so, but still an ultra! Lairig Ghru is a race from Braemar to Aviemore taking the most direct route over the beautiful Cairngorms of Scotland. It scales beautiful hills to begin with before following a rocky valley which eventually leads to a forest and then on to the roads of Aviemore. The start line for this race was a driveable distance from my house so I wouldn't have to rely on the terrifying system that is public transport. This all seemed very sensible. And here, my friends, is where the sensible stops.

Try imagining how you might go about preparing for your first off-road ultra. Got it? Well, now forget it.

I managed to, except remove from the equation any off-road training runs, any time spent learning to read a map or indeed time spent buying a map in plenty of time, and, lastly, neglecting to purchase any decent trail shoes. At best it was a very unique approach to preparing for my first off-road race. At worst it was bloody stupid. I trained on roads for the three months between the Glasgow to Edinburgh and Lairig Ghru over what I thought were plenty of hills. I would come to learn in the months that followed Lairig Ghru that these were not proper hills, but that's for another chapter. For now, these hills were enough for me to find challenging.

I bought the map required for the minimum kit list two days before the race and didn't even open it. I estimated my current road shoes had enough miles left in them and would just be careful where I put my feet. This would mean trail shoes shouldn't be necessary; I mean, it was just going to be a bit bumpier than a road race with a couple more hills, right? It didn't even cross my mind to Google the route, look at pictures of the route

47

or even recce parts of the route during those 12 weeks of training. Sigh.

The sunny, late June morning rolled around and I felt pretty good. A bit like a puppy at the top of a water slide when I think of it. Completely and sadly oblivious to what was about to happen.

It was a buzzier, more excited field of runners on the start line than those I had come across at the Glasgow to Edinburgh race. Numbers were high enough to create an atmosphere but still low enough to make the race feel close-knit and comfortable.

We set off, and during the first section of the course I kept hearing mention of a boulder field coming up at some point. This sounded interesting and definitely more exciting than 55 miles of canal. Bring it on, I thought! When a stretch of the valley came into view, littered with rocks for a good two or three miles, I naturally assumed this was the boulder field. Picking my way through this at a stilted jog, I was helped along by a man in front whose foot falls I could follow. Unfortunately, and hopefully not because he was distracted by an annoying girl following him, he tripped and fell a mile or so later and urged me to carry on while he walked.

Reaching the end of this rocky section and beginning a scrubby climb, I felt quite chuffed with myself! I'd managed to stay upright through more than half the course now, still had energy in my legs and had conquered the boulder field everyone had gone on about. And in road shoes! High, five, Shauney!

I crested the hill I was climbing, passing two or three rocks nearly my size before pausing to look up at what was to come next on the course. I blinked a couple of times and squinted at the view again. Boulders. Real, proper, ice-age-esque boulders piled atop one another with no visible flat ground beneath them and stretching as far as the eye could see.

Ah, fuck.

As it turned out, those boulders went on for six miles. Bit bumpier than a road race? Oh, the naivety. But what I lacked in off-road training I had made up for in mental-grit training. At one point about midway across the boulder field I could see no one in front and no one behind. Had it not been for the fact that there were sides to this valley and I knew I just needed to keep going straight through it, I probably could have convinced myself I was lost. It was during this stretch that I thought about some of the crappy training runs I'd had. One of which had been quite recent and had been so utterly dire I had turned to my trusty blog for some reassurance.

June 2016

I think I may have hit rock bottom. Let me explain:

23 miles was planned for this morning, starting at 3am and hoping to finish at 7am. That's not unheard of for me

since it's difficult to get a run done in the evenings with work, horses etc, so it wasn't a big deal.

Up and dressed at 2.30am, I wasn't fully awake but I always think that's for the best — I usually just flop out on to the road in my trainers with bleary eyes and am too tired to put much effort into over-thinking it!

The first couple of miles were a little grating: 'Okay, could do with being in bed just now but that feeling should go once I get into a rhythm and cover a few more miles. I mean, it's getting lighter as I go, and I've run in worse conditions,' I thought to myself.

The five-mile mark comes around and I'm getting more bleary-eyed and my legs aren't feeling too fresh. Well, shit, can't I just have a nice, easy long run today?!

By the 6/7 mile mark I was light-headed, tired to a ridiculous extent, no energy worth-a-monkeys in my legs and my thoughts were getting darker. Even the banana in my backpack couldn't drag me up out the slump. I know right! It was that bad!

9 miles: I ground to a complete standstill. For 90 minutes or so I'd been thinking about the charity and the work they do which is great but I kept coming back to how little my running campaign is doing. I'm trying to get myself to Everest to run there in order to raise awareness and funds, and yet one day on a cake stall can raise almost as much as the last eight months of 3am starts, sweat and injuries. I'm not an ungrateful person

— the donations so far have humbled me and I was over the moon every time one came in.

But my thoughts this morning had gradually turned into: what the fuck is the point? This isn't helping anyone. Nobody really cares. Why would they? They're not getting anything out of it. And if nobody cares, no money's getting raised and nobody's benefiting at the charity.

So you see, with no one really paying attention, no one taking the time to wonder what this is all about and how they could get involved, and not all that much support going on, I flagged.

I cut the run short at 13 miles. This is something that really got to me because I never quit, but I just could not keep going. I admire other fundraisers who keep a great big smile on their face, never seem to lose their motivation, raise thousands of pounds and make the whole thing look effortless.

Of course, I'll bounce back, my energy will recover, and I'll be a chirpy, annoyingly motivated, headstrong fitness freak again, determined to make her fundraising work a success very soon. But right now, I'm going to sit here, with my tea and toast and jam and consider how miserable I can realistically make myself.

For now, I'm signing out, the moody runner.

It gave me some solace to know I didn't feel as bad as I had that day; my mind was clear if somewhat strained by the prospect of such rough terrain, and my overall outlook was good, all things considered. I would manage to pull myself through this drastic section of the race, and I'd be absolutely fine. But as an aside, who looks at that terrain and thinks: I can barely walk over that so let's make people race over it? Bloody sadists!

By the time I crossed the line in five hours 48 minutes, my shins and knees had handed in their resignation and thoroughly disowned me. I hobbled to the free food tables, more concerned about the disappointing fact I never felt like eating when I ran, even though the post-race meals are totally included in the entry and usually plentiful. Goddammit, I thought, spitting out the mouthful of cereal bar I had attempted to eat. My stomach told me where I could shove that idea.

For my first attempt at off-road racing, Lairig Ghru had been successful, but only really because I'd gritted my teeth and not because I'd been remotely prepared. It had been a learning curve more than anything, but sadly not enough of a learning curve, as I would discover in the months that followed.

Chapter Six

Shakespearean tragedies and swearing at the sky

July 2016

It was going well so far and the first parts of the plan to get to Everest had actually come together, much to my amazement.

And so, being the impatient person that I am and undoubtedly beginning to feel a little overconfident, I decided to batter on with the next part of the plan: I started looking into the hill racing scene. I quickly learned the grades and types of events and found a Grade A long hill race was the toughest I could aim for. Did I start small and build up to this? Did I heck. I entered an 18-mile Grade A hill race, just two months away in the Scottish Borders. I had just done a 28-mile trail race, after all! A few more hills over these two months and I'd be totally ready for an 18-mile hill race. This was my slightly deluded thought process.

Two months later

It wasn't to be, let's put it that way. Hill runners reading this will roll their eyes and most likely glean a very slight hint of satisfaction when reading the rest of this. The Two Breweries Hill Race was to start in Innerleithen in the Scottish Borders, cresting some of the most majestic hills in the region.

Driving down first thing in the morning, I began to get a little jittery as we reached the Borders. I've visited the area before and have always thought of the misty, romantic hills as being dramatic and fantastical; a sight to spark the imagination. They weren't quite so fantastical this morning. They were big. Really, really big. I hadn't trained on anything like this! But these weren't the hills we would be tackling, I reasoned with myself. The race organisers wouldn't be that cruel, surely? I will always, always have to learn things the hard way, it seems.

We arrived at the correct car park in plenty of time but this did nothing to quell the feeling of doom beginning to creep over me. Once I'd registered and pinned my numbers on, I sat in the passenger seat of the Shogun, watching the grim, grey sky and a variety of stringy-muscled, short shorts-wearing, serious-faced individuals completing an interesting array of warm-up routines. They were, perhaps, even more intimidating than the Glasgow to Edinburgh bunch! There wasn't a single person here who looked out of their depth. I probably would have felt more at ease stepping off a spacecraft on Mars than stepping out of the car that morning.

Standing on the start line for the race briefing, I think it began to dawn on me just how slapdash and wing-and-a-prayer my preparation for this had been.

'Oh fuck, oh fuck, oh fuck,' was all that was going through my head as the steward counted us in and shouted 'Go!', and the field belted off at, in my lowly opinion, a stupid pace. I set off at my usual pace (which felt like a plod amid this lot) and left my stomach somewhere far behind. A part of me must have known what was to come.

I was beyond inadequately prepared, of course. I had been correct in my thinking on the start line. I was surrounded by machines. Absolute, 100 per cent, machines. But if I'd thought, even for a moment, I might have actually been adequately prepared on the start line, the sight of the first hill would have erased that thought. These were the hills that made up the *backdrop* to my usual hill runs. I didn't think anybody was stupid enough to run up them! As I slogged in slow motion across the top of one of the early but still ridiculously exposed hills, marsh up to my mid-calf, leaning at a 45-degree angle against the driving rain and gales that had started over an hour ago, I considered the kind of idiot you had to be to do this on your Sunday off. A certifiable one was my conclusion.

After mounting those early hills, we began to creep closer to the real hills – the ones that gave this race its Grade A status. They were bigger and crueller than even those I'd seen during the drive down here, I'm sure.

I just was not ready for the severity of them. Like, at all. I had thought, very naively, I would be able to power up a section at a time, catch my breath and regroup on the downhills and the flats and be ready for the next steep climb each time. Think again, Shauney! The downhills were shockingly steep and took almost as much work to get down as they did to get up. As I slid down a good few metres of one, on my arse, I considered it might be easier to just lie on my side, give myself a shove and roll down at speed. And the flats? By the time I reached the top of Huddleshope Heights, where you could say it was a lot flatter, I could barely stay upright against the wind and rain.

One checkpoint later, the marshals were lying down, peeking out of their hoods, probably willing me to move goddam faster because they desperately wanted to go home! I reached 11 miles, two miles after the point I had decided to pull out, soaked to my knickers even through waterproofs, something close to tinnitus in my ears, and hands frozen to the shape of the map case I was carrying. 'Flip this for an idea' (or words to that effect) was all that was going through my head and I gratefully, if not gracefully, retired.

I wasn't alone: 18 of us retired from the race, but even without the terrible conditions I would have been hard-pushed to make the cut-off times for each checkpoint. Hats off to the runners who power through these races and manage them in shockingly fast times. Just then, I couldn't see how I'd ever be one of them.

I obviously pulled out at the nine-mile point but alas, this was too far into the middle of absolutely nowhere for a pick-up vehicle reach. The next point at which the route touched the road wasn't for another two miles. During these two miles, I and another runner who had decided to pull out tried to pick our way down a treacherously steep hill made up of marsh, clumpy grass and an obscene number of rocks. I removed my map case from my left hand and my hand remained frozen in the same shape, it was so exceedingly cold in the wind. At one point, I thought I should at least try to make the most of the views. You know, something about being on a hill in the wild Scottish Borders seemed classically romantic and something to be enjoyed. I lifted my head in a vague attempt to look up at the view and almost lost my face. If ever an expression could be fixed on your face by the weather, this was that moment.

Even running meant taking both feet off the ground for a split second, which turned out to be dangerous in itself. I'm not exaggerating here as I was stupid enough to try, ending up on my hands and knees two feet away from where I was supposed to be. Being the eloquent lady I am, I shouted, 'Fuck off! Just. Fuck. Off!' at the sky at that particular moment. The other runner just a few metres in front of me didn't even hear me, because of the storm in his own ears.

Two sweep vehicles picked up a wet, sorry-looking bunch of us from a farm building at the 11-mile mark. Once dropped off at the finish line, I traipsed back to the Shogun like a shivering, half-drowned rabbit looking for somewhere to curl up and feel sorry for itself.

My grand plan to reach Everest seemed to have veered off the tracks, along with my confidence. It had shocked me how hard I had found these hills, and if I couldn't do a few hills in Scotland then how was I supposed to run a marathon on Mount Everest? It was a pie-in-the-sky idea and, despite my previous delirious belief that it might be possible, I had realised with an almighty crash back to reality that it wasn't. Not for people like me anyway. The Everest Marathon was an elite race for elite runners. I wasn't anywhere close to being an elite runner. I wasn't even in the same district, country or universe, for God's sake. I'd been a little girl, with little-girl ideas, and I'd just found out Santa wasn't real.

Chapter Seven

Sheep whispering

The mental battle of trying to convince myself I would be able to run one of the toughest marathons in the world in 2017 was finally lost. I let go of the idea of doing it so soon, allowing myself to come around to the concept of looking after my mind and body rather than torturing myself over miles and trainers and rocks and shin splints. The deadline for entering the 2017 Everest Marathon was December that year and there was no feasible way of gaining the experience I still needed before then. And I didn't want to.

The marathon was run every two years, meaning the next one would be in 2019. I would aim for that one.

Having to pull out of the Two Breweries Hill Race meant my confidence was now in tatters and I wanted to hide away. And with my mind now shifted to the 2019 Everest race, that's exactly what I did. I turned my back on the Run Watson Run campaign, on race training and on the whole idea of being mentally driven towards the goal I'd been so sure of. It sounds so stupid when I look back on this period of time now. After all, people pull out of races all the time. For me, however, it meant I'd failed at something I'd been only just convincing myself I could do. I thought I'd learned failure growing up, just like everyone else, but this was stinging! I'd been burned and I didn't want to put my hand near the flame again.

I didn't post on my blog, I didn't look at races I could do, I didn't write up training plans like the slightly manic person I usually am. I wrapped myself in the strange security of the gym. For me, it was hiding away. I buried myself in working away on the weight machines. This was without much improvement, it has to be said, as I'm no weight-training expert! I got busy swimming as many lengths as I could each week. I spent far too long wrapping myself in knots on the total body resistance (TRX) straps. However, I will admit the TRX straps are a lot of fun!

I still ran, but random distances, as long or as short as I wanted. If anyone asked, I would tell them I was training for *something*, I just didn't know what yet. This gained me more than a few curious looks.

In reality, I needed the regular kick of exercising but I was shying away from commitment. On the other hand, as most commitment-phobes will tell you, playing the field can be quite enjoyable. I took long runs through the city, people-watching and nosying as I so often like to do. Yes, I am aware I have the mentality of an 80-year-old sometimes. I love the countryside for its beauty but sometimes the city is just way more interesting. For instance, when you're running in the countryside, you would never come across a fluffy-pyjama-clad woman marching up the street at eight o'clock on a Saturday morning, screaming down her phone in one hand, cigarette hanging from the other. Believe me when I say the stories you can conjure from that image can occupy a good half hour of any run.

However, the time did eventually come where I emerged from hiding having licked my wounds sufficiently. I began to run a little longer, keeping my legs in good working order a little more and thinking tentatively about races I could possibly do. Only possibly, though! Looking back, this period of recuperation had come at exactly the right time: I'd put so much constant pressure on myself as I trained for Glasgow to Edinburgh and Lairig Ghru. I never let up! Even while friends and family gave me concerned looks and told me to ease up on myself, I had obsessively kept going. I was desperate to prove something to myself. And though my training had often been misguided, it had always been hard, spending nine to ten hours a week training, with six of those spent running. For an amateur runner with no professional training, this was a hefty schedule.

Scurrying away and hiding from this recent failure actually gave me space from my own obsessive mind, and time to gain a new perspective.

Perhaps my first 'lift' from this recuperation spell came when I found the hill at Balintore.

When I was a child, my parents moved our family out to Lintrathen, a tiny village at the foot of the Glens. My mum had grown up in the Glens, with her dad being a shepherd. Moving back out here was returning home for her, and my brother and I spent many years being told stories and shown places she used to know.

One of these places was Balintore Castle. I remember, at eight years old, being driven up to Balintore Castle to see its sad, decaying remains. Mum told us of the beautiful, grand castle that had once stood here. It had been built in the 1800s by a politician who had been made rich by his family's investments in the East India Company. By the 1960s it had been abandoned, sadly, due to extensive dry rot. It then passed from person to person, slowly slipping further into disrepair. In 1994, the castle was bought by a Taiwanese businessman and hopes were raised among the locals that the castle would be restored to its former glory. Unfortunately, the years went by and the castle continued to fall to pieces. After years of objections, the council finally managed to compulsorily purchase the castle and it was then bought by its saviour – a gentleman by the name of David, who has been slowly restoring the beautiful old building since 2011.

The castle sits amid the rolling hills of Glen Isla. There is a winding country road – usually teeming with rabbits and skirted by deer – all the way up to it. Driving up for the first time in many, many years I was taken aback by the beauty of the castle on the side of the hill in the distance. It was almost enough to bring a tear to my eye, seeing it being restored to its former grandeur.

Parking my car a little away from the castle and surrounding cottages, I decided I was going to explore this place. It was a place which inspired me with its beauty and peacefulness and I guess part of me was starting to itch again. Running for fitness like a normal person was all well and good but I'd made a promise (to myself more than anything) and that wasn't going to lie dormant forever. So I was up here with a baseball cap and a pair of trainers in search of a different kind of run. And in my usual haphazard way, I found a track that led to a hill which then led to a *hill*.

March 2017

'Oh ya ******.'

The words I uttered when I reached the bottom of the hill I had vaguely seen on Google Maps. The '475m elevation' on the trusty little online route planner hadn't really meant much when I read it on a screen. Shading my eyes as I squinted up at the very distant, very high hilltop, it meant a lot more now.

Wheezing my way up the previous (much greener) hill, I had been oblivious to the extent of my unwise choice until this point.

For some reason, despite running for about four years now, I'm still clueless about distance. I was certain the top of the nice green hill would definitely be as far as I had planned ... and I definitely wouldn't have to climb that massive, massive hill starting to come into view ... even though this path looks like it joins that paa ... oh bugger ...

Day one: I can't lie. I got to the bottom of this big, heather clad, rocky beast, looked at my watch and went 'Yup, tea time.' I promptly turned around, and I didn't even feel bad.

Day two: (yesterday) I told myself to suck it up and put my brave girl pants on. My poor quads would just have to feel like they'd been through a mincer for a bit, but you can't seriously expect to be able to be a trail runner without some sore muscles. I mean, get a grip woman. So up I went, cursing the sheep who seemed to motor up it effortlessly in front of me.

I stopped and started my way up to about two-thirds or maybe three-quarters before stopping properly. Well, long enough to hear something other than my own wheezing anyway. All while giving myself a verbal telling-off for being so unfit. I live in the countryside, in Scotland for goodness sake, why isn't this a doddle? Anyway, what I heard when I stopped needing an ambulance ... was hardly anything at all. Being on my own, this high up and this far from civilisation was the quietest thing you can imagine. Birds calling in the very far distance were the only sounds to be heard, and that in itself made the shaky legs worth it. And this being a beautiful clear day, the hills around me and the views right across Angus were breathtaking. That's if you have enough breath left to take of course.

I clambered back down the hill, which may well have been as tricky as coming up, and made my way back to my car, set on the idea of doing this hill as often as it takes to get good at it.

Day three: (today) 'It's half six in the morning, what in Christ's name do you think you're doing, you absolute lunatic,' is what I'm sure the sheep were saying as they watched me half drag, half trip up this same bloody hill, obviously looking so pathetic it never even crossed their minds to run to safety. I'd have to look like a potential danger to them for that to happen. Even the little gammy-legged one was thinking, 'Bring it on, love.' But I got to the top this time! And my God, the views were even more worth it. Looking out over the other side of the hill, you can see right over to the desolate, snowy mountain tops, steep ravines below, and cliff faces making the landscape look wholly prehistoric. The wind was whipping over the heather around me. It's a strange thing, being in the middle of such vast, immense, empty hills, and what it can do to you. You feel completely alone, insignificant and tiny. Not in a bad way, just in a very blunt, truthful way. A sort of realisation settles on you, and you're not sure if you feel really, really at one, or very spaced out. Or perhaps the exercise is getting to me.

I almost wet myself when a grouse came hurtling past making an ungodly racket. Clearly, I'd been standing on top of his hill long enough.

I will be back next week, to undoubtedly amuse some more sheep and hopefully find I can do considerably more running rather than sitting on my arse cursing my unfitness.

For now, signing out, the incredibly hungry runner. Like, seriously, there's not enough food in the supermarket to satisfy what my body thinks it needs right now.

And there it was. I'd ignited my spark again. I had a buzz and a fixation again. These few hill runs turned into regular training. I wanted to be able to do this! With the spark ignited, and my confidence beginning to at least build if not be totally restored, I started to look for my next race a little more seriously.

It had to be one I felt, with enough training, I could actually do. But it had to be challenging enough to catch the Everest 2019 race organisers' attentions.

After considering a few, but with none of them really jumping out at me, I finally found the Ultimate Trails 55km trail race in Ambleside in the Lake District. Now, I'm going to admit here, the main reason I opted for this one was not for its terrain, elevation, qualifying points or technical challenges, because I didn't really look at any of that. It was mainly because it was 55km so my fundraising text line 'HBUK55' (after HorseBack UK), created when I first planned to do Glasgow to Edinburgh's 55-mile race, still made sense. Oh, will I ever learn? This particular race was the shorter version of the Ultimate Trails 110km, and I guess this made me feel comfortable with it as it was the 'novicey' option (ha ha ha).

Both this race and the 110km, if completed, were worth three and six 'UTMB' points respectively. Whatever they were.

Chapter Eight

Death by seagull and other fatal circumstances

April 2017

With Ultimate Trails 55km booked and a comfortable three months away, I began to feel excited at the prospect of being back on track for my Everest campaign. I had till 2019 to get the experience I needed, and this ultramarathon seemed like a sensible step towards that.

But this feeling of excitement was different to how I'd felt about races before. I was used to the mix of excitement and nerves, but this was excitement with a core of anxious cautiousness. I'd been knocked down after thinking I could achieve something last year, and it wasn't beyond the bounds of possibility that it would happen again.

But I was learning. I knew I had to learn from past mistakes and push my training further and harder in the right direction if I wanted to do bigger and tougher races.

I couldn't just run lots of miles and hope for the best now. I had to be more organised and strategic in my training. I was up to my hill at Balintore at least twice a week, working harder at cross-training in the gym and taking at least one rest day as well as a long-run day and recovery-run day. I was basing my training around two hard weeks followed by one light week rather than constantly trying to up my mileage week after week. Training hard, I had learned, required sufficient healing time and that was non-debatable.

My actual running skills were starting to improve at Balintore – I had a stronger gait and suffered fewer injuries – and I was now constantly on the lookout for hills, as steep and as long as I could find for my hill-training days.

May 2017

I went on my first long (ish) hill run the weekend before last which went surprisingly well. As in, I only got a tiny bit lost as opposed to a big bit lost.

Sunday came around and, much to my partner's never-ending, alarm-induced misery, I was up and out the door at four o'clock in the morning. I parked up at my start point at around half past four and set off, still a tad sleepy, but not at all lethargic.

I had planned my route in the most easy-to-follow way possible. It started on a track anyway, so happy days for the first mile or so. When it came to leaving the track I was, not for the first time, reminded Google will never be able to tell you the current livestock status of a field. As in, this one was full of Highland cows. I think I'm just drawn to them. I never seem to fail to end up in among them, despite efforts not to.

Anyway, they were standing a good bit away so I figured I could dash to the other side of the field quickly enough for them not to bother with me. And this would have been fine had it not been for the small river and the fact I had forgotten to put on my waterproof socks. I didn't fancy getting wet feet at this early stage so I figured I'd just jump it.

Except the spot where I needed to jump from was sunken and sloping and not great for taking off like a little gazelle over the water.

Overseen by the cows who most likely rolled their eyes and continued chewing on their cud, I took a couple of very un-gazelle-like runs at said river, only to chicken out and build myself a little path with rocks to cross it instead.

Cursing myself for being such a wuss (when do I ever chicken out of anything?!) and the cows for laughing, I set off up the hill on the other side. Trying to locate the right track took far longer than it should for someone planning to do a trail ultra in just a few weeks, but with only a couple of extra additions to the route and only a little swearing I managed to locate the right track on the right hill!

I must have reached the top of this heathery, rocky hill around 5.30/6am and apparently seagulls have a very big gathering at the top of this particular hill at that time on a Sunday morning. I started to freak myself out by noticing they were only flying en masse above this hill, and furthermore: only above me. This was it. Death by seagull air stampede. If anything's going to make you move faster, imminent death by seagull will.

I reached the other side of the hill in double quick time, climbed a fence and found myself looking out over the most beautiful valley Angus must have to offer. Being this time of the morning, I disturbed a herd of red deer who took off, looking glorious with the morning sun on their coats, and a couple of hares shot away from me as I paced down the steep side towards a farm and a road. Or at least I hoped there was a road, otherwise I was in completely the wrong area.

Now, despite Google showing a track from the bottom of the hill to the road, it failed to mention the field of sheep I needed to cross. At this time of year, I seriously doubted any farmer would be chuffed at his lambing ewes being frightened by a rather dim-witted runner. However, after skirting along the surrounding gamekeeper tracks, I couldn't see another way so, very carefully, I shimmied along the track through the field, telling the sheep in hushed tones to keep very still, don't make a sound, I would be gone soon (yes, I am an utter weirdo, I know). And just so you know — they were all pretty cool with having an intruder sneak through their field at six in the morning.

All was well and dandy until I reached the farmhouse and the farm dogs decided to raise merry hell. I got my arse into gear and got out of the vicinity before a farmer came out with a shotgun.

The majority of the rest of the run was hilly but on road surface. By the time I finished the 14 or so miles, I can't say my legs felt too fresh but overall, it wasn't a terrible reaction to my first longer hill run. I finished up in front of the gorgeous Balintore Castle, currently being restored to its former glory, and that, with the views across the tops of the hills, made my Sunday complete.

June 2017

The nice kickback from seeking out steep, long hills to train on is finding some of the most gorgeous, undisturbed places almost on my doorstep.

Very early one morning, just a few weeks before the Ultimate Trails race, I drove out to the walkers' parking area near Loch Lee in the easterly region of the Angus Glens. The scenery around me was just becoming visible at this time of the morning. The ragged and rolling hilltops several hundred metres above me were still dark silhouettes in the grey light as I wound my way along the twisting country roads to the car park.

I stepped out of the car, breathing in that sharp air that tells you it's going to become a clear, beautiful summer's day, and pulled on my baseball cap. I warmed up (I was learning!) on a track that ran perpendicular to the path leading to the loch, and then headed off at a contented jog, following the signs for 'Mount Keen'.

The path ran fairly flat for the first three miles, crossing little burns and winding its way to the mouth of the hills. By the time I crested the first of these hills the sun had broken above the horizon, diminishing the early morning grey, and casting the deep valleys and rolling hilltops in a glorious, rich light. It was so silent and so beautiful I stood for several moments smiling like an idiot on the side of one hill. This was what it was all about.

There was a little more climbing before Mount Keen at 939 metres came into view. This was to be my first Munro run and, despite being in a wonderfully good but rare running mood this morning, to say I wasn't doubting my decision would be a lie. (A Munro is a Scottish mountain over 3,000 feet high, named after Sir Hugh Munro, who first listed them in 1891.)

Mount Keen is the most easterly of all the Munros and seems to rise very quickly out of the rolling hills. At the time, it looked a smidge too much of a challenge for my off-road, in-training legs, but I'd come this far; I might as well give it a bash. By the time I reached the summit, legs beginning to scream as I picked my way over the piles of grey and green, lichened stones, the beautifully still morning some metres below had given way to a relentless, battering wind that came and went over and over in sudden bursts, much like the tide.

Up here, it was wild and exposed with not a living creature in sight, and yet from this point you could see 360-degree views for tens of miles, which was incredible. However, the wind was terrifyingly ferocious when it picked up, and dulled my sense of hearing and sense of touch, which is why I felt inexplicably vulnerable from all sides. The heebie-jeebies ran through me like nobody's business! I ducked behind a wind block of some piled stones, so I at least had my back to something and could enjoy the views to the west without feeling like the honey monster was about to grab me from behind.

To be honest, I'm the same with hand driers: if I have to use them instead of paper towels I have to put my back against a wall or have a mirror in front of me. Clearly, I'm supposed to work in the secret service.

Here I was, completely alone and crouched behind a windbreak on top of a small Scottish mountain, a mix of adrenalin, rushing blood, inexplicable fear and giddy excitement coursing through my body. I felt alive! Really, truly alive! Mount Keen is described as the bleakest of all the Munros. Maybe when comparing photographs it is, but when you're at the top of this Munro, completely on your own, with miles of hills below you, it is an awesome place to be in every sense of the word.

I was trying to take in the immense views, smother the flighty part of me which wanted to get out of here as fast as possible, and quell the massive grin on my face because it was giving me druggie-high giggles. Between the conflicting excitement and nervousness, I was becoming aware of how cold my limbs had suddenly become and that, along with the tidal-like battering wind there was also cloud coming and going around me. Approximately 90 seconds after this realisation, I couldn't see more than about 20 feet front of me and the wind was no longer coming and going. It was constant. Viewing time was over and the fact I was an amateur on these hills, on my own, with no mobile signal and limited map skills was suddenly very stark. Thankfully, I had noted the marked guidance stones on the way up and I could just about see from one to the next until I was down lower than the cloud and into the silence again.

It had turned from eerily beautiful to scarily powerful quicker than I had expected, giving me a definitive reminder that proper hills were not to be underestimated or treated in a blasé manner. They were real and dangerous and, much like the sea, should be treated with caution.

Chapter Nine

The technical way to not fall off a cliff

Ambleside, Lake District, 1 July 2017

As far as perfect racing days went, this sunny morning at the beginning of July in the Lake District was shaping up to be one. Or at least a spectator at the start line in the luscious, leafy park would have said so. However, with the current feeling of total and utter doom that had, yet again, settled over me, I wasn't so convinced. I had spent the entire drive down to Ambleside the day before muttering phrases like, 'this is such a bad idea' and, 'why didn't you stop me when I first mentioned it?' to my exasperated, long-suffering partner. The drive alone seemed doomed as our usually robust Mitsubishi Shogun kept overheating. By the third stop to let it cool outside a service station, I was convinced the entire race was cursed. I watched a young couple strolling past, laughing without a care in the world, service station coffees in their hands. I could see nothing funny about the situation.

When we finally began to approach Ambleside we joined a road I knew would be on the first leg of the race. We were driving it in the opposite direction to the way I would race tomorrow, meaning the 13 per cent downward gradient which went on and on was all set to be tackled uphill on foot the following morning. And this was at the very start of the race! Oh dear.

I wasn't sure what to expect at this stage to be honest. I knew not to underestimate the squiggly lines on the course-profile map. Especially not the three massive peaks among them. It didn't comfort me that this first section we were driving was not one of those peaks on the map.

Aside note: check me out reading the course profile before the race and everything! But anyway.

I registered when we finally got to the village and had my kit checked. There was a queue winding between two tables for this, and buffs and numbers and the like were handed out. The queue was full of serious-looking runners and I was impressed that I didn't feel as intimidated as I might have 18 months ago, although this was probably only because I managed to further convince myself that the race marshals wouldn't let me through the registration. I couldn't think of what it was I had forgotten but given the near disastrous journey here, I must have forgotten *something*. I have not been gifted with the most logical mindset as you may have gathered. Ambitious yes, logical no. For this reason, I was amazed that they finished checking my kit without a hitch, let me through to get my number and wished me luck for the forthcoming race. I wanted to say, 'Really, are you sure? Are you sure I've actually got everything?' I did have, apparently.

The next morning came around and I can't say I was massively nervous. It was too late to do anything but resign myself to the fact that there was a significant chance (or so I thought at the time) I'd be driven back in a mountain rescue vehicle by two o'clock that afternoon.

The fact that the race didn't start till 11am meant the beautiful, cloudless summer's day could take hold and make me fret over the heat starting to build. Goddammit, I'm from Scotland! We don't do heat!

We started off through the village of Ambleside, which itself is on a hill, before passing through to the quiet country roads beyond. The scenery was immediately idyllic, and I was even able to appreciate it a little between worrying about the heat and how steep the hills would get. The first leg was called 'Struggle to Kirkstone Pass' and had been the section we had partly driven the day before. It was tough because it was steep and I wasn't used to the heat but otherwise the terrain was fine with half of it on road, and it was over more quickly than I had expected.

The second leg was more technical underfoot and a lot more downhill, both of which I really enjoyed, and it reminded me of why I prefer trail to road running. Keeping upright was challenging both physically and mentally which ate up the time, and we were soon at the second checkpoint. By this time, I was starting to think, 'Oh, hang on, there's a chance I might manage this thing ... maybe.' But I knew from the course profile that the biggest and apparently toughest climb was after checkpoint two, so I attempted to psyche myself up at the feed station, which thankfully had a queue in which I could stand and rest. I was very impressed with the facilities at this checkpoint: the spread was fantastic, not that my stomach would have withstood anything strange I put in it, but I could appreciate the effort. They also had real toilets! REAL toilets!

Anyway, that's beside the point. We started climbing as soon as we left the checkpoint and the terrain began to get a little rockier. The views were incredible as we reached the top of one of the first smaller hills, over a stunning, sparkling lake with the sun still beating down. It started to get cooler from this point as we continued to climb. The hills, however, were not as bad as the ones we all knew were coming. We finally reached a point in the valley with gargantuan sides and it was a guessing game as to which one we would negotiate to get over and out. None looked appealing to be honest.

I dealt with the eventual steep, rocky climb by talking to a few folk. One man had done this race two years ago and another was doing it for the third time. You meet some of the craziest people on these things. By the time we got to the top, the weather had changed to light drizzle which was fine by me. We skirted a lake you could only get to by foot, and scaled another, shorter climb before the treacherous descent to checkpoint three. I think I know what 'technical underfoot' means now. It means 'suicidal'. I had learned my lesson from Lairig Ghru and my sticky first hill race and had trained on proper hills for this event, but nothing quite as dangerous as this descent. Some runners had poles, which I'm still dubious about. However, one kind man did lend me one for a section where a slip would have proved fatal, and I have to say I didn't die so maybe there's something to be said for them!

I was still enjoying myself at this point as, unlike other races I had done, the field hadn't spread out to total lonesomeness. There were still a handful of folk to run with and talk to and it rallied me along nicely.

There was set to be another climb after checkpoint three but it was 'just a little one' according to the course profile and anyone I asked. They all lied. It was hideous. Let's not even go there with that one. This was probably the start of the mentally-tough part. Once I had finally got over that hill and to checkpoint four then came the *much*-longer-than-expected leg to checkpoint five. 'Just around the corner,' I kept thinking. It wasn't. It really wasn't. The views were still pretty, the terrain was still challenging but the race was turning into a real mental slog. The field had spread out a little more by this stage and I did spend a fair amount of time on my own with my own darkening thoughts.

My feet, legs and back were hurting. My toenails ... well, let's not go there either. I'd been running and climbing for almost eight hours by this point, and all I wanted was my bed. I was pretty tired.

Even when a marshal finally came into view and said, 'the checkpoint isn't far; just behind the school', he also lied. I couldn't even see a building, let alone a school! There was a teary moment at this point, and a 'for God's sake, Shauney, pull yourself together, woman!' moment, but eventually checkpoint five did appear. The atmosphere at this checkpoint helped to encourage me. Every runner was sore and tired but willing to give a fellow race participant a few words of support and some distracting conversation. The marshals were excellent, and as I left the checkpoint, I felt rallied.

There was one last climb before the finish which, after nine hours of running and climbing, wasn't the prettiest section of running I've ever done. Although, by this point we were coming across one or two runners coming to the end of the 110k race, and the pain on their faces made me feel ever so slightly better about my own circumstances. My blisters could have been so much worse!

Despite this last hill, the very last little section was a delight. And that's not even sarcasm! It was all downhill and for some reason I had imagined the finish line to be a lot further away than it actually was. It appeared quite suddenly and the utter joy I felt at that moment meant I managed to bounce across the finish line with a big smile on my face, in a time of nine hours and 42 minutes.

We were served up an incredible choice of post-race meal options which smelled and looked to die for but, as is always the case after miles and miles of running, I couldn't even swallow a bit. This was definitely the most disappointing thing about the day! I went to bed with an exhausted but contented smile on my face a couple of hours later.

If you've ever done an ultramarathon or long-distance endurance event that lasts for several hours and then tried to go to bed straight after, you'll know what my sleep felt like that night. You have this sudden realisation of what an incomprehensible effect so many hours of physical stress has on you. My entire body twitched all night, and my dreams were lurid and fitful. My period had started by the morning even though it was nowhere near due, and it's not until you step under the shower that you realise exactly how much skin you have lost as you scream every swear word under the sun when the water hits you and sears all your raw flesh. But part of you is slightly satisfied at the fact you have managed to push your body to such a state it has these involuntary responses ... once the painkillers have kicked in the next morning, of course.

As it turns out, despite my inane ability to belittle every training effort I make in my head, I *had* trained enough and my body *was* ready for 55km of technical trail, even after a cursed road trip to get to the start line.

The relief I felt in the days after this race was far greater than when I'd accomplished anything before. So much had rested on completing those 55 kilometres. First and foremost was my self-respect. I needed to test myself and see if I was strong enough to learn from my previous mistakes and complete something seemingly impossible while my head was in a place of such doubt.

The inner voice that had been putting me down for the last nine months could now just shut the fuck up! I had three 'UTMB' points!

These, now I'd actually Googled them, were qualifying points for Ultra-Trail du Mont-Blanc. So that explained why it was so technical and why the hills were so lethal in parts. But it made me grin from ear to ear to realise that, though I had found it challenging, I hadn't struggled!

And so, I had renewed hope now. The pie-in-the-sky idea had been lassoed and pulled a fraction closer. I had a little more faith in my physical abilities and now reckoned I probably could train for the Everest Marathon. But where to go from here? I had ultra experience, I had trail experience and I was starting to get my head around hill running. What did the Everest race organisers expect now?

Chapter Ten

Out of the frying pan

Just before Glasgow to Edinburgh, over a year ago by this stage, I had attended a talk about the Everest Marathon which, quite coincidentally, had been held in a town just an hour or so from my house. It was organised by a group leader from the Everest Marathon in previous years. I had kept his card in the hope I would need it one day.

I found it in the crease of my wallet a few weeks after the Ultimate Trails race, well worn from being carried around everywhere. Obviously, some part of me had held on to the stubborn belief that eventually it would be useful. I had been wondering and wondering what on earth I was going to do now. What else did the Everest race organisers need to see from me in the coming year to be accepted into 2019's event?

Eventually, I concluded, the only thing I could do was speak to an organiser or leader of the race so they could advise me.

I phoned the number on the card, hoping the line still existed, and waited for an answer. The conversation that ensued left me a little breathless. Somewhere between butterflies and knocked off your feet by a frying pan to the face.

As it turned out, the ultramarathons I had already completed over the course of the last 18 months, and the trails and hills on which I had finally proved myself was enough to grant me entry to the Everest Marathon *this year*. But this was the end of July and entries for the 2017 marathon had closed in December 2016. I pointed this out to the group leader. He informed me there were still a couple of places left (cue butterflies) and, though it would be a tight window in which to get everything organised, if I was quick at getting my paperwork to the organisers I would likely be accepted (cue frying pan).

Despite my excitement at the prospect of running the marathon at Mount Everest this year, it was a big decision to change my mind from the 2019 race to the one in just four months' time. My initial thought was, 'I'm not good enough yet. I'll be good enough in 2019 but I'm not good enough now.' However, after a few words from my dear mum it occurred to me how incredibly well I undermine myself at every given opportunity. I think it's the same for most people, especially in sport.

She told me I should read over my previous blog posts as they seemed to make out I did very little to train for these races I 'foolishly' signed up for and that it was a miracle I'd completed any of them.

'Well, this is true!' I said. 'I really don't do nearly enough!'

She helpfully reminded me of the hundreds of hours I'd accumulated on the roads and hills over the past two years; the stupid o'clock starts I'd had some mornings just to fit in a marathon-length run before work; the pain and frustration of being injured and having to start it all again; not to mention the tedious cross-training thrown in between.

I started thinking about this. I read over my previous blog posts and found she was right! I was undermining my efforts at every turn, more effectively than any abusive trainer ever could!

Just got back from a 20-mile run before breakfast? All very well but I had to walk one hill!

Had to take a week off? Laziness! Never mind the miles I'd done the previous week!

Completed a race I believed impossible? Fantastic, but how on earth will I manage it again? So I gave myself a mental slap and told myself to stop being such a stupid cow.

I'd trained successfully for the seemingly impossible before, hadn't I? And anyway, it wasn't like anything was going to be different between now and 2019. I may have done more races by then but chances were I'd have the same level of fitness and a lot less money! My conclusion: 'Suck it up, buttercup, you can do it this year, so you're doing it *this year*,' I told myself sternly.

Of course, my physical ability wasn't the only factor that made me doubt the decision to run the 2017 race. While a normal entrant for this race had from January to organise themselves, my entry was accepted at the beginning of August, a mere three months before we were due to fly. I had just ten weeks to get my vaccinations, flights, medical certificate, Nepalese visa and essential kit organised, not to mention making arrangements for work and horses to be taken care of. Six of those weeks I had to find corporate sponsors who would fund the trip.

I still can't tell you where those three months went. By some miracle the funding was pulled out of the bag by some very generous companies and individuals just in the nick of time; all my paperwork was in order by mid-October.

Halloween Night 2017

It's Halloween and the trees and landscape here in Scotland are all in oranges and browns, a feeling of nostalgia settling over the hills as summer becomes a memory. And so too does the summer of training on sometimes scorching, sometimes wet and wild hills and trails.

> I fly to London in a week's time to join the Everest
> Marathon crew and, though never entirely confident in
> my training, I think I've done all I can to prepare. There is
> just one last thing I need to assure myself I can do.

At this stage, I was oblivious to the fact that we would have a team of wonderfully talented porters with us who would erect our tents at each campsite. I thought this would be entirely my responsibility. Having never had sole charge of a tent before, I decided it was high time I learned.

My perfectly formed plan was met with dubious concern from my partner, friends and parents. Apparently, it would be wiser to pitch a tent in the garden and figure it all out with a kettle and kitchen on standby.

Well! That is just not the way I do things, people! No, no, I would drive myself out to the familiar car parking area a few miles from Mount Keen, trek with tent over my shoulder and all essential kit in my rucksack to the foot of the mountain and camp a night there. In the morning, I would take a training run up the Munro before packing up and trekking back to my car. What could possibly go wrong?

In hindsight, checking for a suitable area to pitch a tent prior to trekking out in the dark may have been advisable. Familiarising myself with the tent-building instructions may also have helped. And checking the weather forecast. To be honest, there were a great many things I should have checked before hauling the unreasonably heavy rucksack and tent on to my back and traipsing off in the pitch dark this Halloween night. My trainers, rolled-up Therm-a-Rest and tent were all strapped to the outside of said rucksack and swinging around something hellish.

To begin with I found the idea of doing this on Halloween quite funny. It was the cliché opening to a horror film waiting to happen. But as I traipsed onwards, the moon moving in and out of the clouds and animals rustling in the undergrowth or skittering under rocks, I began to make myself jump. And then, as I began to move up off the low-lying track, out of the shelter provided by the hills and into the valley, the wind picked up and started to whip around me so that I couldn't hear anything. By the time I reached the spot I figured I'd probably be able to pitch the tent, I had convinced myself I was being stalked by a faceless axe-murderer who would grab his opportunity any second. Why was I doing this again?

After three miles with the stupidly heavy rucksack weighing me down, my shoulders were aching and the wind was starting to slap my face raw.

Unfortunately, the spot I had considered might be usable (based on a vague memory of the area when I last passed it a few months ago) was all heather and rocks and on far more of a hill than I would have liked. On the other hand, it was starting to rain now and I was getting pissed off. This spot would have to do.

With much swearing, I managed to unpack the tent. Pinning the flapping fabric under one foot and holding the torch between my knees, I unfolded the completely useless instructions and tried to convince myself I had control of the situation.

It took me a full hour to construct something I could climb in and zip shut. Note: it looked nothing like a tent. By the time I piled myself and all my belongings inside, the wind and rain had turned to full-blown-howler status with sheets of rain battering the already flaccid tent fabric. I was soaked but remaining stubbornly in denial about the complete disaster around me.

I lay in my sleeping bag for all of five minutes before the front A-frame fell in on me. I continued to lie there. It was waterproof. It would be fine. I just had to fall asleep for a few hours then I would wake in the morning, go for my run and then never speak of this again. It was fine, I repeated over and over to myself through gritted teeth.

I lay there for two hours, determinedly refusing to let the wildly flapping tent fabric and completely collapsed frames change my defiant camping-experience plans. That was until I felt the icy prickle of water seeping into my thermals. I shot upright and found myself sitting in a deepening puddle of water.

'Oh, just fuck off!' I shouted skyward.

'FINE!' I pulled my clothes back out of the stuff sack in a strop, still sitting in the murky puddle of water. Attempting to re-dress myself, my head acted as a tent prop for the sodden fabric more than anything else. I stumbled out of the mess and back into the storm with wet feet and arse, hurriedly trying to repack everything substantially enough to get back to my car. I had no idea if half my stuff would eventually end up lost forever on the heathery hillside. The tent, I'm fairly certain, still isn't in its casing correctly. I haven't gone near it since the unfortunate incident. I learned a valuable lesson on packing that night: don't do it in a storm at 1am. To relay the stream of swear words that left my lips during the course of the very soggy walk back to my car would fill a chapter all by itself.

I glazed over the details when my slightly smug relatives and friends asked how it went, knowing full well I had returned, soaked to the bone, at 3am.

'Oh, you know, worthwhile experience and all that,' I coughed.

November 2017

Packing my kit bags had been a challenge in itself because of an exceptionally tight weight restriction for the flights on the short take-off and landing aircrafts we would be boarding to Lukla airport in the mountains. Despite these weight limits, we still had to be prepared for two weeks of extreme heat and cold, hiking and running. My cat had watched on with mild bemusement as I stood, hand on head in my living room, muttering to myself amid stacks of clothes and equipment, trying to decide how much I could strip away.

It was a bit of a blur but, nevertheless, on 7 November, I found myself sitting on an Edinburgh to London flight, diary on lap, not sure whether I was fully prepared or had forgotten almost everything. As we flew out of Scotland, I wrote:

I'm not entirely certain how to convey the excited-anxious-buzzing-dread filled-startled-stressed-pinging off the walls feeling I'm having at the moment. It's a bit confusing. Having been focussed on this challenge for precisely two years and the cause it's for, I'm now faced with it imminently. It was never imminent before! It was always a far-off idea that any sane only-done-one-marathon runner would have sensibly considered too far out of their reach to achieve. But my addled brain persisted with the far-off idea, determined to prove some sort of point (to myself probably). But that's what it remained: a distant date. So now I'm in the twilight zone I guess. It's really just a wing and a prayer now. The whole thing is an unknown quantity. Running 26.2 miles after trekking for two weeks at -20 with ice, rocks and ridiculous drops, and 50% less oxygen than my body needs? I could be magnificently ready or completely fucked. I really have no way of telling.

Over and out, the neurotic runner who shouldn't be allowed to make decisions without adult supervision.

Chapter Eleven

Into the fire

I guess the point it all started getting very surreal wasn't when I decided I wanted to run a marathon at Mount Everest or even when my entry was confirmed; it was when I was sitting at the back of an old, faded bus travelling through the streets of Kathmandu three days before we were due to fly out to the Himalayas themselves. When I say 'travelling', what I actually mean is being thrown from side to side as the driver expertly, if not comfortably, weaved in and out of the masses of trucks, cars, bikes, people, horses and tiny three-wheeled buses packed with locals. He'd slam on the brakes, blare the horn and then speed off again the very second a gap in the chaos opened up. It reminded me a lot of the Knight Bus from Harry Potter.

It was dusky at this point in the evening as we were being transported from Kathmandu airport to our hotel, and I was somewhere between trying to fight off the urge to fall asleep after the long flight and frantically trying to take everything in. Nowhere was quiet; the city was a constant babble of people, traffic, blaring horns, ramshackle buildings, piles and piles of electric cabling bunched around posts and looping down on to the road, random cows, chickens and goats, and so many motorbikes!

Despite it being dusk, the small bus was sweltering and the beautiful necklaces of flowers our very kind driver had given each of us were giving off a pungent aroma. I felt as though I had been picked up and thrown straight into a film. Every sense I had was suddenly heightened and intoxicated! I'd seen images and programmes and movies like this, set in India or Thailand where some traveller or national or spy is making their way somewhere important and exotic, but I'd never considered it all to be real. And while I had been living my same, old Western life, watching these films, it was all actually happening! All this traffic and bustle and commotion; trade, poverty and riches; overcrowding and under development, and yet lives being lived amid it anyway. It's satisfyingly startling to be shown something so contrary to what you are used to and what you so often take for granted.

As stupid as it sounds, all I could think was, 'I'm on a bus in the middle of Nepal!' It was a very strange sensation. Then the bus driver realised he had missed the turn-off to our hotel, slammed on the brakes again

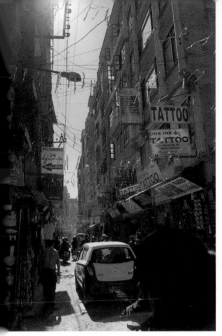

The bustling, chaotic city of Kathmandu was a barrage on the senses

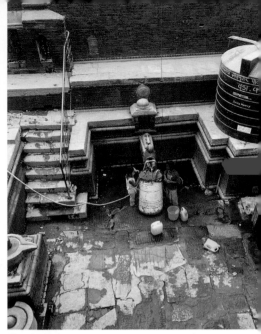

Basic living arrangements round every corner

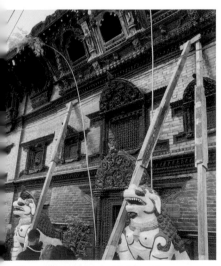

The damage caused by the earthquakes of 2015 is still evident today

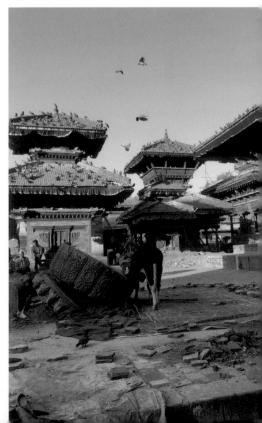

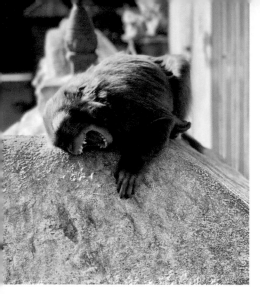

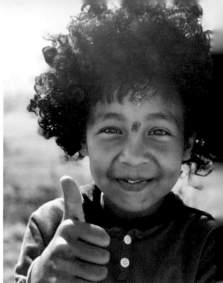

A tired resident of the famous Monkey Temple in the Kathmandu Valley

The locals were delighted by our wigs and costumes during our 'fancy dress training run'

Our first glimpse of the majestic Himalayas

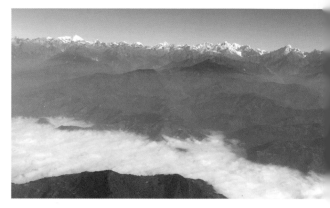

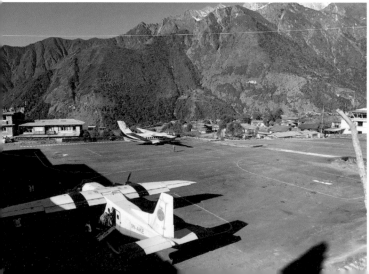

The infamous Lukla Airport (Tenzing–Hillary Airport) where the runway can be seen disappearing over the cliff edge

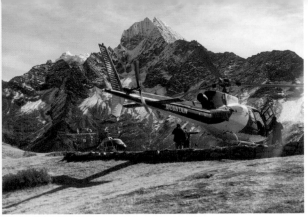

Helicopters are prevalent in the Himalayas

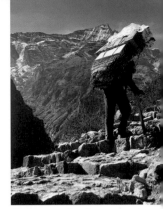

Porters take huge loads in their stride

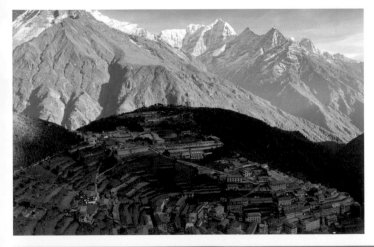

[Left and below]: The trading village of Namche Bazaar, carved into the hillside

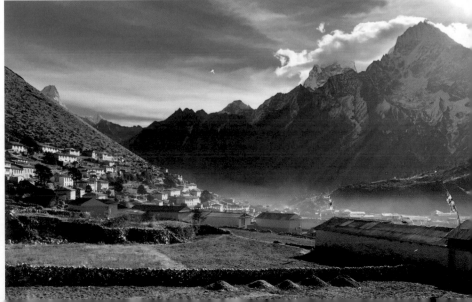

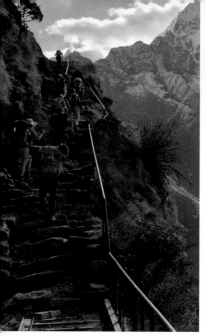

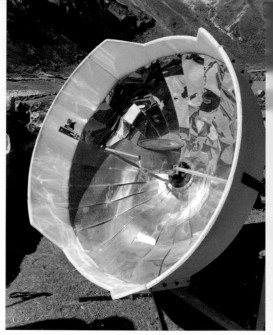

The breathtaking trek
gets underway

The Sherpa way of life with ingenious
tricks to make the harsh lifestyle that bit
easier. This device heated water during
the hot days

The rope bridges we would
become accustomed to

Two dzos in front of one of the many
prayer wheels dotted up the trail

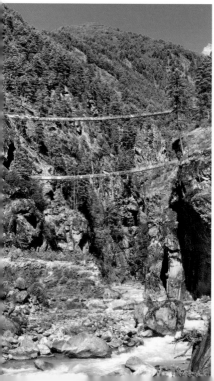

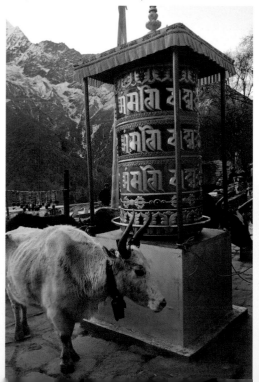

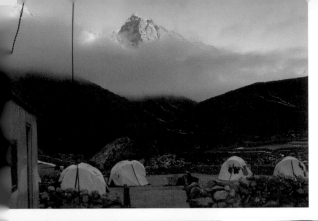

Our camp at the village of Machermo

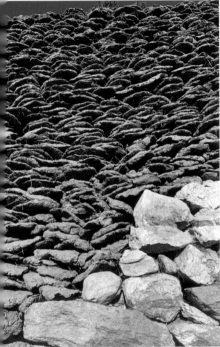

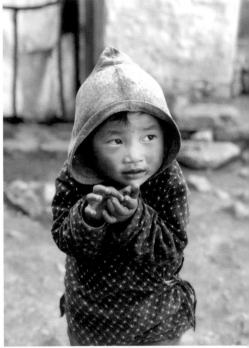

Piles of yak dung, drying in the hot daytime sun, ready to be burned during the freezing nights

One of the many friendly, charming Sherpa children we came across

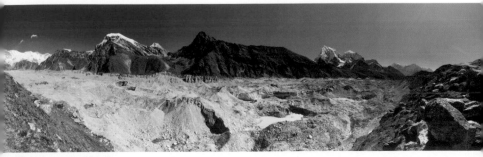

Ngozumpa Glacier

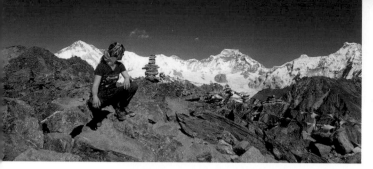

At the summit of Gokyo Ri, with Everest just out of the photograph

At the summit of Gokyo Ri, looking over the famous Gokyo lakes

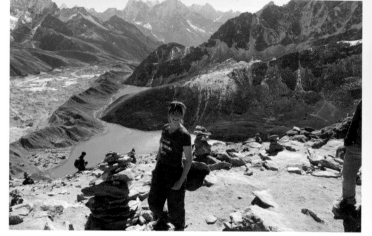

One of the buildings in front of the stunning Tengboche Monastery

Three of the memorials at the Memorial Ground for fallen climbers

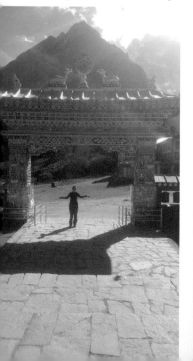

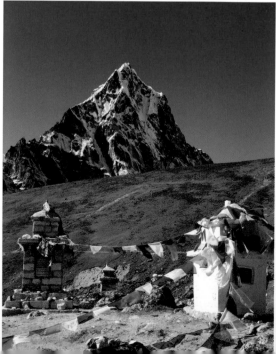

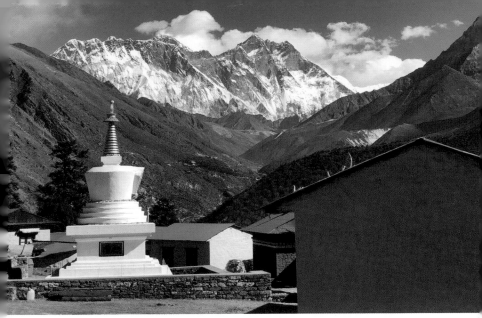

Tengboche watched over by Everest itself

Creeping closer to Everest, the terrain becomes tougher underfoot and gives us a taste of what the first half of our race would entail

Only a few miles from Everest. At this altitude, pure yaks were used on the trail

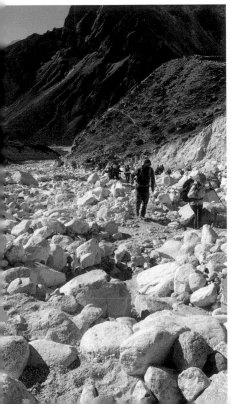

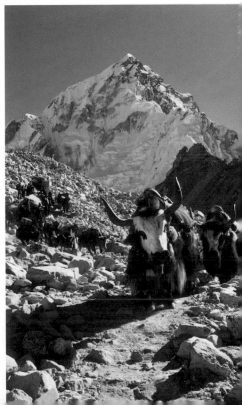

At Everest Base Camp, in front of the Khumbu Icefall where mountaineers and potential Everest summiteers begin their climb

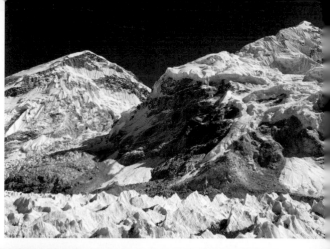

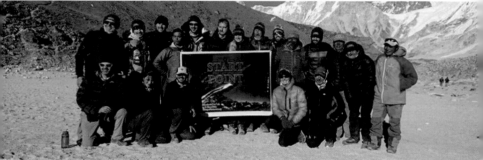

On the start line the afternoon before our race, just as I began to feel queasy

Neema, our kind, humble and incredibly strong guide

Crossing the finish line and giving way to relieved, exhausted tears

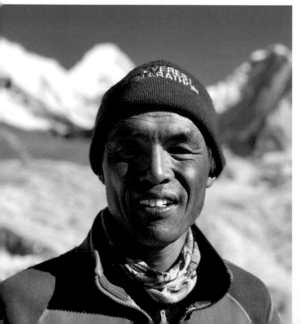

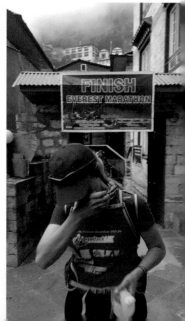

and swung the vehicle across ten 'lanes' of traffic. Lanes would suggest there was some order in place which there really wasn't. He swung the bus in a U-turn back on itself and we all clung on to our seats and looked at each other with slightly panicked expressions. You could say the race-participant bonding started early on this trip!

11 November

I'm sitting in a hotel room in Kathmandu. This all still feels like a parallel universe. We fly out to Lukla tomorrow and I am quite beside myself with anticipation. I have no idea what the next few weeks will hold. The only thing I know is that by the end of it I will have had the biggest adventure of my life to date. To be on the cusp of something as exciting as this is slightly surreal but utterly incredible.

For now, we're staying in a former palace set in front of beautifully kept gardens and a sparkling pool. It's amazing and certainly adds to the bizarreness. In three days' time we'll either be sleeping in tents or very, very basic lodges with no toilets. It'll be a world away from what we're used to. In fact, this hotel is a world apart from the city it sits in. With its spectacular gardens, clean and decadent interior and peaceful atmosphere, it couldn't be further removed from the shambolic, bustling city.

Experiencing the streets and villages of Kathmandu is incredible. It seems so far from Western living with priority on functionality more than aesthetics. You can see where the Western world is trickling in, though. Advertisements seem to indicate being white is a good thing. Partying and dressing fashionably is what should be strived for. I saw a box of Russian vodka in a liquor store window with the slogan 'happy water for fun people' above a picture of some partying young white people. I found it quite sad. People in this country look at people from the Western world and strive for our pointless infatuation with clothes and drink and 'beauty', while we look at them and envy their wholesome lives. Here, you grow food, you sell it. You carve wood, you sell it. You learn to work with your hands and a value is placed on that. Of course, this is a generalisation. Nepal has a growing technology industry, and the UK has a wealth of talented tradesmen. But there's not the same legislation, and health and safety, and red tape here in Nepal. If something needs doing, they do it. If it doesn't need doing, it doesn't get done.

It was pointed out to me that Britain too was once a developing country and went through all this pollution, disorganisation, poor quality of life, etc. But I wonder if Nepal will end up where we are now in a hundred years' time. Part of me thinks not. Advances in technology seem to have been put in place here before organisation has really come about. Electric networks, for example, are in complete disarray. This was something we never had to contend with.

It put things into perspective. For me anyway. It's important to remember that the values and priorities you have at home would be completely different on another part of the planet, so are they really worth getting hung up on?

Being a young woman who had travelled very little in her life, experiencing such a different culture to my own flipped my perspective around every time I saw something new. It seemed to be a constant, humbling game of mind-shifting and realisation.

I was running through a small village out in the farming province of Kathmandu dressed as Peter Pan (let that sink in ...) and I got that surreal 'what-am-I-doing?' feeling again. We had a training run on our itinerary for early this morning and to help us get to know one another we were running in fancy dress. This was, of course, far more to do with providing amusement for the locals than anything else. The villagers ranged from being delighted by the stream of Westerners dressed in ridiculous clothes running through their villages to downright bemused.

The children, with very little in the way of material things or entertainment in their lives, were overjoyed to see these strange characters passing their houses. The delight on a small child's face when he was given a tartan bonnet with ginger hair attached was touching.

And the groups of children running to windows or out on to the street to wish you 'Namaste!' was a glimpse of the innocence these young people grew up with. They likely had no televisions or computers to get any sense of a world beyond their own village. Their village was their world and perhaps that was more real than the computer-generated, media-driven world we so often find ourselves wrapped up in.

What I found interesting was the amount of political turmoil and, to be frank, downright drama in Nepal over recent years which we hear little to nothing about.

Direct rule from a king ended in 1951 after the beginnings of political unrest. A succession of prime ministers then became the leaders of Nepal. The monarchy returned briefly in the 60s but the government soon regained power. It was during the late 1900s that political unrest started to become more prevalent. The most turbulent of which has been in the last 20 years, with violent protests damaging buildings and costing lives.

A massacre of the royal family in 2001, when Crown Prince Dipendra shot nine of his relatives before turning the gun on himself, marked the beginning of the abolishment of the monarchy altogether. Reigning for just two days while he was in hospital with what would eventually be fatal wounds, Dipendra's crown passed to his uncle, Gyanendra.

Gyanendra ruled until 2008, during which time he faced constitutional turmoil and eventually decided to hand over control to the Nepalese Constituent Assembly, which abolished the monarchy completely. Nepal is currently run by Bidhya Devi Bhandari, the leader of the Nepal Communist Party and the country's first woman president, though it remains beset by disputes, unrest, repression, corruption and oppression.

It seemed to me that Nepal, with all its high-energy bustle, exotic culture, hidden gems, political turmoil and the unrest of the population as a whole just recently, was being quite overlooked by the developed countries which really should have known better. How many other places were there like this in the world?

Chapter Twelve

Puddle jumpers and cliff-drop landings

Being the wonderfully disorganised person that I am, I hadn't actually looked into the mode of travel we would be taking to the Himalayas when I first decided to do this marathon. I didn't even look into it when I applied, for that matter. It wasn't until a month before I flew to Kathmandu that I sat down to read about some of the finer details of the trip.

Our trek started 80 miles from Nepal's capital and, as pretty as the Nepalese countryside was, I don't think any of us would have relished the thought of trekking that 80 miles or indeed taking the day-long bus.

Instead, we were due to fly. This sounds all well and good until you quite innocently Google 'Lukla airport', the airport we were flying to, and consequently end up reading through a list of the 'most dangerous airports in the world', on which it features rather highly.

Google Images didn't offer a much better response, with one picture showing a plane in a very smashed-up condition against the side of the mountain, after the airstrip had been misjudged by a pilot in conditions that had suddenly become adverse. The picture had been taken earlier in 2017. I closed that web page and vowed not to tell my mother about this.

Sitting on the runway one month later, waiting for the safety checks to be completed on our plane, there was no web page to close. I considered that I could probably stride up the side of this puddle jumper with wings in four or five steps, while the 'safety checks' were akin to the kind I do on my car: quick kick to a tyre and a nod to the pilot.

The airport man chaperoning us on to our plane stood at the front of our bus and announced in limited English (though not as limited as my Nepalese):

'Very strong people at front of plane; rest at back.'

We exchanged quizzical expressions around the bus before someone piped up, 'By strong, do you mean the fatties?'

'Yes,' the man nodded, clearly glad he was communicating with us effectively enough. 'You, you, you and you at the front.' He pointed at four or five people before disappearing to help pack our bags into the hold.

It was most amusing, because of the fact that none of us were particularly fat. Some were just slightly broader or heavier-set than the slight Nepalese figure. Nonetheless, fatties to the front, lightweights at the back. I ended up somewhere in between, staring out of the little window and feeling distinctly like I was sitting in a tin can. Despite this, I was excited. I figured I was flying on this plane regardless of how I felt since there was no other feasible way of getting to Lukla in time. I could either enjoy the hairy-scary ride or sit petrified in my seat. If it did crash into the cliff face beyond and below the end of the runway then the result would be the same regardless of how I'd felt during the ride, and at least I would die doing something exciting.

With steeply ascending ground at the northern end of the 527-metre by 30 metre, 11.7 per cent gradient single runway, and a steep drop at the southern end, it's not difficult to see why Lukla airport is often listed as one of the world's most dangerous.

Sir Edmund Hillary, who was the driving force behind the airport's construction, had originally wanted it to be built on flat farmland but this became impossible when the local farmers refused to sell any of their land. The strip of land the airport sits on now was bought from local Sherpas for $2,650, and the same Sherpas were employed to build it.

The runway was only paved in 2001 and was bare ground before this. Apparently, at the time of building the airport, Hillary bought some local alcohol for the Sherpas and asked them to perform a foot-stomping dance on the airstrip to flatten the soil and provide some resistance for landing and take-off.

In 1953, Hillary and Sherpa Tenzing Norgay were the first people to summit Mount Everest. During the course of our expedition it would become clear just how much Hillary cared for the Sherpa community, and how much he had invested in it. His legacy is still apparent and has continued to help the community since his death in 2008.

There were accidents at the airport in 1973, 1991, 1992, 2004, 2005, 2008, 2010, 2012 and 2017. The worst was on 8 October 2008 when 18 passengers and crew were killed after their plane hit the airport fence and crashed into the steep cliff face below the runway before bursting into flames. Camera footage shows heavy cloud over the runway at the time of the crash. No flight is permitted to take off from Lukla in poor weather conditions and pilots must have confirmation of clear conditions at Lukla before departing from any origin airport. However, the weather in these mountains is notoriously changeable and some flights can be caught out, forcing pilots to attempt to land in poor conditions.

The difficulties faced by pilots at Lukla airport mean strict guidelines are in place, which stipulate the experience required of pilots permitted to land at the airport. A pilot must have completed over 100 STOLs (short take-off and landings), have over a year's STOL experience in Nepal and have completed ten flights or more into Lukla with a certified instructor.

This gave us at least a little faith in our pilot, as we clung to our seats. Excitement was skipping around in my stomach as our little puddle jumper prepared to take off with a lot of noise. It buzzed along the runway and took off into the air with as much determination as I imagine it could muster.

For a while, we watched the terracotta and burgundy colours of the city beneath us growing smaller as people woke up to the usual sunny skies and misty haze lying across the horizon. It wasn't long till we were flying out of the natural 'bowl' in which the city sits. Nepal, many millennia ago, had been a massive lake and when it eventually dried up, a city began to develop in the bowl it left.

I would come to pick up bits and pieces of the history of Kathmandu during my time in Nepal, most of which is steeped in religious folklore, monarchy rule and the Gurkhas.

Dating back to ancient times, as far back as 167 BC, Stone Age tools and a full stone statue from around AD 185 have all been excavated from the Kathmandu Valley. The valley consists of three main cities, Kathmandu, Lalitpur (Patan) and Bhaktapur.

Evidence shows that the lake filled the Kathmandu Valley and, during the time of the first Buddha, had a pilgrimage place at its north end. A Buddhist saint is said to have cut open the southern rim of the valley, draining the lake and creating a huge bowl-like area of fertile land for crops and houses to be built, beginning to create the cities we see today.

Twenty minutes later, we were heading over increasingly larger and vaster hills, forests and terraced hillsides. This simple description doesn't really do the landscape justice. The sheer depth and magnitude of the land beneath us, rolling and soaring, was like nothing I'd ever seen before. Quite literally millions of trees swept out as far as you could see, disappearing into the mist on the horizon which had turned startling white with the morning sun behind. But without a doubt, the most awe-inspiring sight of the morning was our first glimpse of the mountains.

Ragged, snowy peaks sat majestically across a third of the horizon. They were seemingly hundreds of miles from us but still closer than I'd ever imagined myself being to these famous Himalayan mountain tops. This was our first taste of how humbling these mountains were. These structures have stood on Earth – been part of Earth – for 50 million years. They've stood there, inhospitable and immovable, as your high school sweetheart dumped you in the final year, as the Large Hadron Collider was built, as Freddie Mercury died, Neil Armstrong walked on the Moon, two world wars were fought, and during every single major celebration and catastrophe and every unimportant event in the history of the Earth. It makes your own tiny existence feel quite futile. In a way it is both utterly devastating and exquisitely liberating.

It was in this mindset that we caught our first glimpse of the runway we were to land on, through the pilot's window. Yes, we could see straight through the pilot's window from our seats! The Google Images page had not done the airport any justice, or indeed prepared me for how ridiculously miniscule that airstrip would look. It very much reminded me of trying to land a skateboard on half a stick of gum from a hundred metres off.

Thankfully, the morning was beautifully clear and our pilot was more skilled than I will be at anything in my entire life. We landed smoothly on that stick of gum, even if the subsequent seconds involved slamming on the brakes and taking a 90-degree right-hand turn into the 'parking' area to avoid hitting the wall at the end of the runway. I was told, 'It's so much better now they've tarmacked it!' I dread to think of the landings pre-2001.

Stepping off the plane, adrenalin still buzzing through each of us, we filed into the section of the airport building where our bags were being deposited. I couldn't take everything in fast enough. We were here on the edge of the Himalayas and at the start of the biggest adventure of my life.

And for a country girl like me, things were about to get mental.

Chapter Thirteen

How to avoid being cursed

Our fetching purple bags were grabbed from the chaos of trekkers and guides and airport workers, and heaved outside the small airport building. We would be able to organise ourselves better outside the cattle market-like bustle. Once some order was restored, or at least everyone was accounted for, we headed over to a teahouse which offered some relative calm.

Lukla is a small village in the Solukhumbu District of the Himalayas and is the first point reached by most trekkers flying to the region. The airport consists of one small building with everything it needs inside. The short runway and 'plane parking' are alongside. The village surrounds the airport and offers all the basic amenities a trekker could wish for, from cafes and bars to lodges and a bank. Here at the teahouse, we were getting our first taste of Kumbu hospitality with the option of black tea or lemon tea as we sat around a stove and waited for the rest of the group to arrive. As an aside, tea was really rather nice at this early stage. Sadly, I'd be so over it in two weeks I wouldn't want to see another cup ever again.

Maps were being taken out and pored over, talk of routes and what was to be expected on the trail was buzzing around, and queries over how much hand sanitiser we had between us and whether it was likely to be enough were becoming an increasingly regular topic of conversation.

Outside, our purple bags were being loaded on to the yaks. We had first glimpsed them as we made our way over to the teahouse. I say yaks but really these were dzos: a cross between a yak and a cow. Yaks don't do well below 3,000 metres and we were currently at just over 2,500 metres. Apparently, these crosses are better tempered, and less fluffy to boot. Whatever the case, I loved them and vowed to bring one home with me to live out its days with an irritable Shetland pony I knew. This sadly didn't happen.

Once we'd regrouped and organised ourselves we set off, rucksacks on, buffs and sun cream at the ready. It was very much like being at the start of a long run for me. Have I forgotten something? Is this rucksack rubbing? Are my socks slipping? I'm sure I've definitely forgotten something. What am I doing? Oh God, I need the toilet. However, once I stopped over-thinking every detail and actually looked around at my exotic and undisturbed surroundings I was soon so distracted that my socks could have slipped right off and I wouldn't have noticed.

From this point on, everything we saw was new, foreign and exciting. The prayer stones, which are massive boulders perfectly painted with white-lettered prayers, and prayer wheels with their ornate designs were fascinating. Nobody questioned the rule of passing them clockwise. I'm not superstitious but I also didn't want to be cursed this early on in the trip, thanks. Nor did anyone question spinning the prayer wheels three times for good luck. We learned to navigate the yak (or dzo) trains so we didn't end up knocked off the cliff-edge track, and settled into the idea of climbing the many, many, many steps of rocks and boulders as each steep section came up. To begin with, the suspension bridges were the hardest to get your head and body round. With trekkers, dzos and donkeys bouncing across them at each end, you tended to get caught in the middle, legs frozen, staring at the ridiculously steep ravine beneath your feet because you could see *right through*. After four or five crossings, however, you got into the swing of bouncing along them and ignoring imminent death beneath you.

By the time we reached our spot for the night, the group was buzzing with conversation. For me, the most exciting sight, besides the mountains, was the startlingly blue river we had crossed and were now staying next to for the night. It looked like a children's story-book river, painted a lurid, unrealistic colour. I couldn't stop staring at it! I had frantically tried to get as clear a picture as I could on my camera when I'd first spotted it, oblivious to the fact we'd be pretty much following the thing for the next two weeks.

That evening, a group of us headed down to the beautiful, cold rapids after our first sweaty day in the mountain heat. Being straight off the Himalayan mountain range, the water was sharper than any I'd felt in Scotland, even in the depths of winter. It sent what felt like shards of ice through your blood if you left so much as a toe in for too long. It delighted us all and began the stream of memories we were going to create together over the coming days.

I didn't know why, but, despite being so very far from home doing something outrageously ambitious I was unsure I was even capable of, I didn't feel lost or alien or unsure of myself. I felt comfortable. Perhaps it was because I was meant to be here or perhaps it was because I'd spent the last year and a half doing things that made me feel uncomfortable and was now, finally, confident with new surroundings and challenges.

Chapter Fourteen

How to breathe

13 November

We arrived in Namche Bazaar today, having spent last night in a basic lodge at around 2,600 metres, a good 800 metres below the small trading village of Namche. The lodges dotted up the trail seem to be basic structures of thin walls and ceiling, though my room-mate and I landed lucky with a room that had a real window and toilet.

The night temperature is certainly vastly different to the sizzling daytime heat but at this height, I can't say it's any worse than Scotland will be experiencing right now. Once we're a little higher, I'm sure the Scots will start to feel the difference!

Our second day of trekking was enjoyable, filled with new sights. The most exciting of which was our first glimpse of Everest through the trees once we had reached the top of one particularly steep climb. We could see it just peeking out from behind the other mountains, looking so ordinary among them, it's bizarre!

No blisters to report as yet and my rucksack straps are still comfy so I am a happy bunny so far!

I saw something very sweet on the trail today as I was coming down a rocky series of steps towards a small collection of blue painted, wooden buildings. It must have been around eight or nine o'clock in the morning, and a small boy, not even the height of my hip, came rushing down the rocky steps past me. He was far quicker than my not so nimble feet could manage. He had a tiny backpack in his hands which he was trying to cram his school books into as he hurried. His smart little school uniform was all done up properly and he must have been sent on his way down the hillside by his mother or father, probably with a flea in his ear for being late.

It reminded me that, although this beautiful place is a huge tourist attraction, it is also home to families, the elderly and children. These well-worn mountainsides host so many lives and stories. Different to our own lives in Britain, Ireland, America and Australia, certainly, but children are still educated, the sick are still tended to, households are still upheld. Though the landscape, culture and traditions are so different to those of the Western world, the principles of all those things that give our society structure do not differ here.

Namche is the gateway for many trekkers looking to follow the trails to some of the most famous peaks in the region, not least Everest. If you have forgotten something for your forthcoming expedition, you will most likely find it in Namche. From trekking equipment, clothing and yak blankets to traditional jewellery, baking and a good pint, the cobbled streets are piled with higgledy-piggledy shops, pubs and bakeries.

The village itself is carved into a mountainside, curving around and creating a dramatic scene when viewed from above, as it looks as if it drops away into nothingness. The buildings are colourful, with different types of bricks and roofs used, and all varying in size, with some new and some old. The earthquake in 2015 destroyed many of the buildings in Namche, and it has since seen new hotels and shops pop up as the people who love and invest in Namche have rallied and put efforts behind getting the village back on its feet.

It was here we would have our last night in a decent bed before the main trek, and it was here we would look forward to stumbling back to for pizza, beer and spicy momos after our marathon adventure.

After our stay at Namche Bazaar, we started the acclimatisation leg of our trek up the Gokyo Valley which runs almost perpendicular to the Everest trail. It was important for us to do this leg of the trek, as marching straight up to Everest Base Camp at this stage would have put our lives in serious, real danger. The risks of cerebral or pulmonary oedema stemming from altitude sickness are all too great at this altitude, and their likelihood would have been several times higher if we hadn't taken our time during the trek and acclimatised properly. Each and every one of us was determined to be on the start line fit and healthy for this marathon and so took this phase seriously.

With mountains on either side of us in the Gokyo Valley, data was non-existent and the Everest Link wifi was super expensive and super slow, so for a full week I had no contact with my family, friends or partner. I began to find this a little difficult as the natural symptoms associated with your body trying to acclimatise started to take their toll. I wanted the comfort of coming home and sharing the day's events with a loved one. It's such a little, simple thing that I had no idea I would miss it so much. And as things got tougher, there were no familiar comforts like a hug from your mum or your dad, and them telling you you're doing well and to keep going.

As we trekked higher up the valley, each day's exertion felt like completing a marathon on legs that had done a marathon the previous day. I had wondered what a lack of oxygen in the air would physically feel like. I was finding out. It wasn't feeling like you couldn't breathe or that you were suffocating; for me it was my muscles feeling like they were under way more stress than they actually were. This was purely because they weren't receiving the oxygen they needed and weren't healing after each day's trek. Headaches were one of the common and natural symptoms of the acclimatisation process. I was lucky enough to only suffer one bad headache near the start of the trek. This was mainly from dehydration if I had to pick a reason. Some people on the expedition suffered skull-crushing, never-ending headaches no matter what medication they took or how much water they drank. Mentally, this would have been tough to deal with along with everything else we were experiencing.

My worst time, and the time I was likely to feel least like I could do this thing, was during the first hour of each day's trek. As we got higher, the morning temperatures became colder and colder. When we started each day's trek the sun was yet to rise above the mountain tops, which meant the air was still freezing. This meant our lungs constricted and refused to take in more than a little air at a time, which is all fine and dandy if you're sitting around all day and not needing much lung capacity. But we weren't sitting around. Most of the treks started on unfairly steep sections, sometimes climbing hundreds of feet in the first hour, and with muscles already screaming for oxygen, a pea-sized lung capacity was less than satisfactory.

Pulling a buff up over my face was all I could do to try to warm the air coming in through my mouth, but even then I still felt like I was going to keel over any second. What was more, after a cold night's sleep, our muscles were stiff and uncooperative, making the experience that little bit more grating.

The terrain was becoming increasingly rough underfoot, not that it had been particularly smooth to begin with. And no matter how many times you were assured 'there isn't much climbing today' there was always a monstrous, rocky climb facing you just when your legs were ready to pack up and withdraw from action.

It did make me wonder, as we finally reached 4,000 metres, how tough it was likely to get by 5,000.

It was, perhaps, during these leg- and lung-busting morning hours, that we felt our deepest appreciation of the physical abilities of the Sherpas around us – both those helping guide us and carry our living supplies, and those we were passing on the trail.

Though I already knew it to be true, it was becoming more and more apparent just how much physically stronger they were compared to ourselves. Our leader, Neema, was a quiet, gentle man who was both admired and respected by all the younger Sherpas in the team. But this serene temperament should not have fooled anyone! At a run, this man was like lightning! After seeing him in action for just a couple of days, there was no doubt in my mind that he could have carried all of our bags to the top of one of the nearest mountains at a thundering run and not even been out of breath. He was simply incredible.

The Sherpas' superhuman qualities have been well documented in the past by mountaineers and trekkers, and it's always been pondered what the exact reasons are for these qualities.

A recent study, led by a team of researchers at the University of Cambridge, was conducted during a gradual ascent to Everest Base Camp. It compared a group of ten lowland investigators and 15 Sherpas who lived in low-lying areas, i.e. those who were not elite, high altitude climbers.

Baseline measurements (samples including blood and muscle biopsies) were taken from the lowlanders in London and the Sherpas in Kathmandu.

Second measurements were taken when they first reached Everest Base Camp, and then taken again after two months at Base Camp.

What was interesting was the fact that the Sherpas' mitochondria, which are essentially the body's battery, were more efficient at using oxygen to produce the muscle stimulant adenosine triphosphate (ATP), which is the main energy that powers our bodies.

They also had lower levels of fat oxidation, suggesting their bodies are better at using resources of sugars. Using sugars is a much more efficient way of generating energy quickly, especially when at altitude.

What was more, levels of free radicals, which are harmful to the body's cells, increased in the lowlanders at altitude, whereas the Sherpas' levels were very low.

But the key difference noted by the researchers was in the level of phosphocreatine in the lowlanders compared to the Sherpas. Phosphocreatine is essentially the backup for when there's no ATP left. In the lowlanders, phosphocreatine levels plummeted after two months at altitude while the Sherpas' levels actually increased.

Of course, research into the incredible powerhouses that are the Sherpa people isn't just for our own fascination and admiration. Scientists are hoping to understand why Sherpas are better adapted to dealing with less oxygen, in order to eventually develop new treatments for those suffering from hypoxia – dangerously low oxygen in the blood.

Chapter Fifteen

Think like a yak

17 November

We're at camp in the village of Machermo at the moment. After leaving Namche we trekked to our first camp in Khumjung – a smaller farming village. After a cold night there we trekked to Dohle, passing the first of the ice rivers and experiencing the first flakes of snow falling as the sun slipped behind a mountain that night. The morning of the trek to Dohle found me with a cold taking hold but thankfully I seemed to have picked up by the afternoon. Today saw us on a short trek to Machermo. I kept a steady pace to keep one man company who was starting to mentally struggle from lack of sleep and altitude. We are now at 4,470m.

The highest point on the acclimatisation leg of our trek was the summit of Gokyo Ri at 5,357 metres. Having been trekking for about a week now, I was fairly unimpressed with the idea of trudging over yet more rocks. What can I say; I'm no Bear Grylls. But I was absolutely determined I was finishing this acclimatisation section. More importantly, I wanted to reach the summit of Gokyo Ri. This was for two reasons, really: one was that I wanted to summit the peak so at least, should the marathon go tits up, I had still achieved something; and secondly, I had heard about the breathtakingly majestic views which could be seen from Gokyo Ri and there was no way I was coming all the way out here and not seeing them.

So off we went. I was only mildly dying for the first hour as we climbed the near vertical face out of the campsite at Machermo, heading for the village of Gokyo. I may be exaggerating but gods it felt vertical.

At 4,750 metres, Gokyo is one of the highest settlements in the world. It is passed through by trekkers climbing Gokyo Ri or visiting the Ngozumpa Glacier, of which Gokyo Ri sits to the west. This particular glacier is said to be the largest in the whole of the Himalayas.

At the head of the small hamlet of stone houses that make up Gokyo, and at the perfect point for catching weary trekkers as they come back down from Gokyo Ri, is a small bakery selling massive slices of cake and brownies. It seems it doesn't matter where you go in the world, if there are walking boots there will also be cake.

From the summit of Gokyo Ri, it's possible to see four of the world's 8,000-metre peaks: Everest, Lhotse,

Makalu and Cho Oyu. With these majestic peaks touching the sky ahead of you, below you is the incredible, startling turquoise Gokyo Lake system. These glacier-fed freshwater lakes make up the highest lake system in the world. The lakes are oligotrophic, meaning they have very low algal production and therefore the waters are exceptionally clear, giving the lakes this surreal, fascinating colour.

The lakes are sacred to the people of both Buddhist and Hindu religions. Around 500 Hindus take a holy bath in the lakes during the Janai Purnima Festival in August. The rest of the year it is forbidden to touch the water.

Despite its beauty, the lake system is naturally extremely vulnerable, lying in an ecologically fragile area. The Ngozumpa Glacier, which lies next to the lake system, channels meltwater into a lake called 'Spillway' which, should it continue to fill, will burst and create a threat to everything in its path, including many Sherpa villages.

Having settled into the rhythm of the trek, we were now looking forward to the day's discoveries. However, when Gokyo Ri came into view around half a mile from Gokyo, it looked disappointingly mundane. Just a big brown mound if anything. It wasn't until I squinted and made out the tiny foot-trodden pathway up the side of it that I realised the enormity of this brown mound. Trekkers weren't even visible!

It wasn't a surprise to find climbing it more than just a challenge. A 'trudge' would be a more accurate description of my footfall during that hour or so. All that went through my head as I put one foot down then the next was, 'Think like a yak, think like a yak, think like a yak ... Jesus, what possessed me to do this ... think like a yak ... I don't even like goddamn hills ... yak, Shauney, yak ... kill me now, just please, ground, swallow me up ...' My footfalls were eventually whittled down to a stop every 100 steps to give me a minute to breathe and remember why this was all going to be totally worth it.

I already knew the views were set to be spectacular from the sight of the sacred lakes we had passed to get here. If I'd thought the blue of the river at the start of this journey was impressive it had nothing on these lakes. They were of the brightest turquoise, if I had to put a colour to them, and were surrounded by hundreds of piles of prayer stones laid out by passers-by. They made for one of the most awesome sights of this trip. Though the pictures you see in this book or on the internet look impressive, it doesn't come close to what the area looks like from the top of Gokyo Ri. With the wind and the chill on your skin, heart racing from the lung-stretching, leg-busting climb, head dizzy from the altitude, Everest away to your left and these lakes in front, nothing compares.

It reminded me of why, despite earlier grumbles, I really did love hills, and why I needed to keep reminding myself of how well you were rewarded when you reached the top of each of them. There's little as thrilling as the feeling we had that afternoon.

Chapter Sixteen

The skilled sport of peeing

During our ascent and later descent in the Gokyo Valley, our longest stay was in the tiny village of Machermo. The usual tactic for acclimatisation is to trek high and sleep low to try to avoid altitude sickness. At 4,470 metres, we were at the highest point we had slept at yet.

When we arrived we settled ourselves in, knowing we were sleeping here for four nights. The plan was to trek higher and come back down for three of the days. Many in the group had already suffered bad headaches, nosebleeds, swollen hands and faces, and sickness and diarrhoea (though the last could be put down to good old traveller's diarrhoea more than the altitude). Sleeping at this altitude would be a big test for everyone.

So far, the worst I had suffered was a cold near the start of the trek and a bad headache from dehydration on one particularly hot day. Dehydration is difficult to avoid at altitude because you expel so much water.

Nobody tells you how much you're going to pee once you get above 3,000m, and, therefore, how much you'll need to drink! I would take one gulp of water and need to pee what felt like six gallons five minutes later. By the time we reached Machermo I was feeling distinctly vacuum-packed from having such little water retention and cursing each evening at the fact I would undoubtedly need to pee several times during the night even though I made a point of relieving myself before I got into my tent. The thought of this was enough to make anyone quite emotional at this stage of the trek. The process of getting up in the night to go to the loo involved so much effort. Step one was removing yourself from the sleeping bag you'd expertly welded yourself into, trying not to touch the sides of the tent because a cascade of ice would undoubtedly coat you and your sleeping tent partner. Step two was getting enough clothes on to brave setting foot outside. As much as I wanted to get into my sleeping bag wearing six layers and a down jacket, I had learned early on that this actually led to a colder and even less comfortable night. The sleeping bag would only work if you wore no or minimal layers. But this meant having to dress oneself in several layers before locating your boots and tent zip to trudge across the campsite to the 'toilet' tent. This was a hole in the ground with a tent put around it. God forbid you forgot your toilet roll and hand sanitiser because that meant a trip back to the tent to rummage around with your head torch, knowing full well the batteries in it would be draining from the exposure to the freezing temperatures. All the while you'd be trying in vain not to wake your tent buddy. This routine was usually completed at least once during the night. Joy of joys.

I did ask one of our group doctors about the need to pee so much at altitude. She gave me an explanation involving (and don't quote me on this, for I am certainly no doctor) an increase in breathing rate from the lack of oxygen in the air prompting the kidneys to remove some of the bicarbonate from the bloodstream, so making it more acidic, which in turn makes you breathe faster to try to dilute the acidic blood, and around it goes. Somewhere in the complicated process, you need to pee ... a lot.

Staying at Machermo for more than just one night gave us the chance to watch the Sherpas and passing porters going about their day-to-day business.

One thing I have noticed about the Nepalese, apart from their hardworking nature and practical sturdiness, is their sense of fun. Sitting here at dinner this evening I'm listening to the cooks and Sherpas and children laughing, singing and joking together. The lady lodge owner came bustling through earlier, making preparations for the cold night ahead while bouncing a toddler on her hip and making funny noises to which he would gurgle, making

> them both laugh. Meanwhile, another girl lights the stove by pouring in petrol and chucking in a lit match! Most of us spat out our tea in surprise and amusement at this!

Our team of porters and cooks always rose early to get our 'bed tea' and hot towels ready for us in the morning, swiftly followed by breakfast. This was usually more tea or powdered hot chocolate followed by porridge, eggs and usually bread or potatoes. It's probably worth mentioning here that loss of appetite is a common occurrence at altitude; I lost mine at 4,000 metres and so quickly went off eggs, bread and potatoes. Especially those covered in garlic! After breakfast, the porters usually packed up and headed to our next stop, arriving before we did. Here at Machermo, however, instead of trekking on ahead of us each day, the porters were able to relax and mingle with the locals. I don't speak Nepali but a couple of the younger porters were definitely flirting with one of the lodge girls, I noted one afternoon!

Most of us took the chance, on our rest day, to do some washing. With just a basin of water to do both clothes and hair that day, I soaped up my hair and most-used garments (those I thought might dry quickly, anyway) in the basin then took everything down to the river to rinse off. A little upstream from me, the locals were also washing clothes in the river, laying garments out on the enormous, glacier-like rocks to dry. We washed, ate and played alongside the villagers. The boys from our two groups got a vigorous game of volleyball on the go at one point, during which I'm sure the Sherpas and porters smashed them.

Being accepted so readily into the lives of the locals, though I'm sure they were very much used to tourists, still felt like a privilege. It's a tough way of life up there with limited power and supplies, but I can't say I saw one grumpy person. Everyone had a smile and friendly 'Namaste!' on their lips, no matter how cold the night had been or how heavy the water-butt they were carrying over their head.

By this point in the trek we had grown to have a great deal of respect and appreciation for the work of our porters and those porters and Sherpas we had passed on the trail.

These guys – we'd also pass women doing the same job – carry enormous loads of supplies between settlings. Our porters carried everything they needed to look after us including an entire kitchen's worth of utensils and masses of food. We had passed porters carrying supplies to lodges: everything from beer to toilet rolls to building supplies, and the sheets of wood alone were sometimes the length of a person. At one point we did see a mattress being carried down a mountain trail on a porter's back and head! These loads usually started off in wedge-shaped baskets but were piled so high that the basket would be dwarfed in comparison. The main weight was taken by a strap that sat over their head, and they walked, stooping, with this weight on their backs, up and down the trails. These were the same trails we were finding difficult with our little rucksacks! We were also wearing good quality hiking boots and layers that allowed us to keep cool in the stifling midday heat. Many of the porters we passed wore jeans and sandals. It's easy to think we've had a tough day at work sometimes but it is nothing compared to an average day for a porter. What these guys do every day and never complain about is more than most of us would ever consider doing in a day. And especially not for the little amount of pay on offer.

On our rest day in Machermo, we met two doctors who were staying a short walk away at an International Porter Protection Group (IPPG) aid post. Each afternoon they would hold a talk for trekkers, climbers and locals in an attempt to educate those attending about altitude sickness and also to raise a little money for the charitable organisation they worked for. They invited us along to their talk later that afternoon, when I learned that the IPPG had been running for many years in this region and that various aid posts and shelters had been built to help the porters who were passing through more and more frequently.

The more they told us about the job of a porter and the, sadly, appalling conditions a lot have to work in, the more shocked we became. We had assumed all the porters we saw were from the Himalayas and were naturally acclimatised. This was not the case. Many were from the lowland cities and struggled far more than even the Sherpas from low-lying mountain areas. I couldn't imagine how torturous some of these climbs would be, carrying the loads the porters were expected to carry, with their bodies struggling for oxygen as ours had been.

These porters can also be massively overburdened and their loads be far heavier than is safe for anyone to be carrying, even more so in these conditions.

The IPPG works to eradicate the avoidable illness, injury and death of porters working in the mountains for the trekking industry. Every year, trekking porters die unnecessarily in the mountains, mainly from altitude sickness and hypothermia, often leaving their families with no income and no food on the table.

We were with a good quality trekking company and our porters wore decent trainers, slept in tents, were well paid and received the tips and clothing we gave them. Unfortunately, not all trekking companies treat their porters this way. Some porters have to sleep in caves at night, in damp clothes with only a thin cotton blanket, while their trekkers sleep in down sleeping bags in lodges or tents. Many are on low wages and never see any of the tips meant for them; overloading can happen all too often. Since the IPPG was formed in 1997 there have been positive changes. Aid posts and hospitals report that most sick porters are now accompanied by a trekker, sirdar or group leader instead of coming in alone.

The IPPG opened a rescue post at Machermo in 2003 which, on our visit, was being manned by these two doctors. They were to stay for three months, after which another pair of doctors was due to take over. Various donations meant they had a portable altitude chamber, an oxygen generator, oxygen cylinders, two pulse oximeters, a stretcher, rescue equipment, solar powered batteries, a satellite phone and lots of medication including Penthrox inhalers.

'The service is free for porters to use while locals have to pay a small charge and trekkers a large charge!' the doctors laughed with us. From this post, a helicopter could take anyone to a hospital in Kathmandu if the equipment on site was not adequate for the condition of the patient.

Knowing a little more about the porters we were trekking with made us not only appreciate them that much more but also realise how much our donations of simple clothing and handy tools meant to them.

Another figurehead to feel strongly about the porters as well as the Sherpas in the Himalayas was, of course, Sir Edmund Hillary. He invested a lot of time and money in making things easier for them and, in time, managed to change the dynamics of Sherpa life quite dramatically.

Born in 1919 in Tuakau, New Zealand, Edmund Percival Hillary started his working life in 1938 at his father's beekeeping business. He was a conscientious objector for the first three years of the Second World War, but a sense of participation and adventure led to him signing up for the Royal New Zealand Air Force in 1944.

His love of mountains led him to the Alps in 1945 once the war was over, and there he learned the ice-climbing skills that would eventually make him the legendary household name he was to become.

Six years later, in 1951, something quite extraordinary happened that may have shaped Hillary's future, and, of course, that of Everest. Eric Shipton, the famous Himalayan explorer, was to lead a reconnaissance expedition to the unexplored south side of Everest. He received a cable from the president of the New Zealand Alpine Club just two days before he was due to leave, asking if he would take two extra countrymen who were currently with another exploration party in the Himalayas.

These two men were Edmund Hillary and the Sherpa, Tenzing Norgay. Without knowing the names of these men, Shipton's instinct was to say no, based on the fact that he hadn't the supplies for extra bodies. But at the last second he changed his mind and said yes, purely because he had fond memories of a previous expedition with another New Zealander. It was during this expedition that Hillary and Norgay put themselves in the running to be picked for the 1953 expedition when they would, famously, become the first people to summit Everest.

Quite remarkably, Shipton had known Norgay before the 1951 reconnaissance expedition. In 1935, Shipton had been putting together a team to explore Darjeeling and from the 100 Sherpa applicants had picked 15. Most of these men were older, experienced Sherpas but one young lad of only 19 was picked because he had a huge grin on his face the entire time, and Shipton had instantly taken to him. This was Tenzing Norgay who would go on to accompany Shipton on almost every Himalayan expedition thereafter, becoming one of the greatest climbing Sherpas of all time.

And so, through pure chance and luck, both Hillary and Norgay would end up on the 1953 expedition led, controversially, by John Hunt. Many thought Shipton should have been leading the expedition but his reluctance to attempt to summit certain peaks in the past had made the Himalayan Committee nervous about choosing him. A Swiss team had very nearly summited Everest the previous year and France had the only permit for climbing the mountain in 1954, so 1953 was going to be the only chance for the British Empire. John Hunt had some experience in the Himalayas and had shown impeccable organisational skills in his previous work as an army logistics officer, and so was deemed the best choice.

The 1953 expedition would prove to be the catalyst for the biggest change the Everest region of the Himalayas had ever seen. Having huge respect and gratitude for the Sherpa people who had looked after and guided them, Edmund Hillary and fellow mountaineer, George Low, felt there must be something they could do to make these people's lives better.

One evening, when sitting with a Sherpa, Hillary asked, 'If I could help Sherpa people, what could I do?'

The Sherpa replied, 'Our children have eyes, but they cannot see. We need a school.' This led to the Himalayan Trust being set up in 1960 and one of its first major projects was to build Khumjung School a year later. Growing from just a two-classroom school in 1961, it now provides education for pre-school, primary and secondary age children and has over 350 students.

The Trust has now built 27 schools and these have been staffed and funded by the government since 1972. This in itself is a major reform. The Trust has also set up two hospitals and 12 health clinics, providing medical support to over 10,000 Sherpas. Through the drive and determination of Hillary and his team, two airstrips were also built in the Himalayas, one of which is Lukla airport, renamed Tenzing–Hillary Airport in 2008 to honour the duo who changed the region forever. The building of the airport made trade and tourism more accessible for the region. In the years that have followed, the Trust has been responsible for setting up Sagarmatha National Park as well as a reforestation project now internationally recognised for the first-class seedlings produced in its three nurseries.

I think it's fair to say that, but for Sir Edmund Hillary and his team, the entire Everest region of the Himalayas would today look very different. Hillary, Hunt, Lowe, Band and Westmacott, all key figures in the 1953 expedition, were responsible for the incredible work of the Trust in the years that followed. They have all sadly passed away now, but their legacy remains, carried forward by family members.

Chapter Seventeen

The monks and the Maltesers

During our ascent, and later descent, of the Gokyo Valley we had stopped at a couple of vantage points to look over at the Kumbu trail in the distance which we would be trekking to reach Everest Base Camp and our start line in several days' time. The most prominent part visible was a ridge we would climb before scaling down the other side. This was around the halfway mark on the trail. Sat atop this ridge we would find Tengboche and, sensibly, Tengboche Monastery.

In the weeks before I left for this trip I happened across a man who had actually taken part in the Everest Marathon in the nineties. It was quite by chance that I bumped into him but also by chance that he had taken part in the marathon that year. We chatted about my upcoming adventure and he told me how he had found it – the trickiest parts and the parts he had enjoyed the most. One particular point he mentioned was a section of the trail where one could enjoy the most magnificent, majestic 360-degree panoramic views of snowy mountain tops and deep valleys. I hadn't realised, while looking back at Tengboche from various points on the trail to Gokyo, that this ridge would turn out to be the spot he had spoken of.

It wasn't until we were standing in front of the breathtakingly beautiful monastery atop the Tengboche ridge that I realised. Around us, the mountains of Tawache, Everest, Nuptse, Lhotse, Ama Dablam and Thamserku felt close enough to touch. The immensity of the views, truly 360 degrees around us, was enough to leave us struggling to find words to describe it. Even now it's difficult to describe the beauty we saw in the middle of that day.

John Hunt, leader of the 1953 expedition, described the sight as, 'one of the most beautiful places in the world. The height is well over 12,000 feet ... it provides a grandstand beyond comparison for the finest mountain scenery I have ever seen, whether in the Himalaya or elsewhere.'

Though I didn't know it at the time, Tenzing Norgay himself was originally from the small village of Tengboche. Since then the village has become renowned, not only for its link to Everest, often being described as the gateway to Mount Everest, but also for its spectacular

Tibetan Buddhist monastery. Tengboche Monastery is the largest monastery in the whole of eastern Nepal and was first established in 1916.

It was destroyed twice, once by an earthquake in 1934 and again by a fire in 1989. The fire, caused by an electrical short circuit, destroyed the monastery's precious old scriptures, statues, murals and wood carvings, though a few books and paintings were salvaged by trekkers. Since then the monastery has been completely rebuilt thanks to donations from all over the world, not least from the Himalayan Trust.

Today, it is something to behold. The beautifully reconstructed building, paintings and carvings and the monastery's setting come together to create, well, something very spiritual.

Mountaineers passing through on their way to attempt to summit Everest are known to light candles and seek the blessings of gods for good health and safe mountaineering. In hindsight, perhaps we really ought to have done the same!

Instead, we sat chatting to the monks in the sunshine, sharing Maltesers, with which the monks were delighted, and generally having a giggle. The group of monks we met were great fun, and one of whom I distinctly remember telling my fellow trekker he had a head like a potato and a nose like an onion – in the nicest way possible of course!

To add to the sensational experience at Tengboche, there is also a teahouse selling the most delicious coffee and cake. What day is complete without good coffee and cake? We left Tengboche smiling with full hearts and fuller bellies.

Chapter Eighteen

The luxury of a tent attracts the wrong sorts

'God's sssake ... too bloody cold ...' I grumbled away to myself, tucking my hands under my arms and burying my nose a little further into my buff as I hurried across the yak paddock. 'Whose bloody idea was this anyway?' I tried to scowl up at the sky but it was a little too pretty to be in a mood with. Nothing but millions of sparkles across a deep, dark velvet, framed by the massive, jagged silhouettes of the mountains we were growing more and more used to every day.

Stamping my feet to try to regain some feeling in them as I reached my tent, I began the high-speed process of trying to locate my toothpaste, toothbrush, Nalgene bottle and thermal bed socks in either my kit bag, day sack or one of the many pockets in my cargo trousers. The time between being outside my tent, fully clothed and grimy from the day, to being tucked up in my sleeping bag (still grimy but wearing fewer clothes) was growing shorter every day. Whether this was down to my improving efficiency or decreasing levels of hygiene and personal care, I wasn't entirely certain.

Grasping the frozen zipper of the tent door, I shook it with just the right amount of pressure to get the thing to open. Nobody could say I hadn't learned anything on this trip. I started digging around in my leg pocket for the toothbrush I could have sworn got chucked in there this morning as I pulled the tent flap back.

'Oh, bloody hell!' I said in surprise, stepping back half a pace. Curled up inside the entrance of my tent was a fluffy stray dog, nose tucked firmly under its tail. 'Really?' I sighed. It lifted its head to give me an unimpressed look. 'Could you maybe leave, please?' I stepped aside and pointed out into the dark, expectantly. If its facial expression could have changed, it would have been to one of stubborn nonchalance. It tucked its nose back under its tail and went back to sleep.

'Fine. Stay just where you are,' I muttered, not particularly wanting to pick a fight with a stray, foreign dog. 'No, no, don't you worry, I'll just squeeze round you,' I said, trying to scrabble around the dog to gather my bits and pieces for the night. The dog didn't even open an eye.

By the time I'd brushed my teeth and stripped off some of my clothes, packed myself into my sleeping bag along with my batteries, phone and camera, pummelled the makeshift pillow of trousers and down jacket into a marginally more comfortable shape, and said a prayer to whoever was in control of my bladder that I wouldn't have to pee six times that night, I was exhausted. And the dog still hadn't moved.

I lay there, clutching my Nalgene bottle of boiling water, thinking I'd truly never known anything to bring me as much joy as a warm Nalgene bottle, apart from, perhaps, the hot towel our wonderful Sherpas brought each of us in the mornings. I began to ponder the mad circumstances I found myself in. I was in a tent in the middle of the Himalayas with a dogged determination to trek every day until I reached our marathon start line. What was that all about? In the two years up till then I'd been so worried I would get my training plan wrong; worried I wouldn't run enough miles, or enough hills or enough marathons; terrified I'd be physically too weak for this challenge.

I couldn't help shaking my head at myself as I lay here in my ice-coated tent. There was no question I was fit enough, and I really needn't have stressed about it all so much. The plan I'd stuck to was more than adequate. The real challenge to this race wasn't really the race at all. It was the environment and the effect two weeks of trekking in this environment would have on a body before putting it through a marathon. In our group alone, there was a whole cocktail of physical symptoms and folk struggling with the altitude, strong sun and freezing temperatures, and we still had five days to go.

Really, I thought to myself, it was more about training your mind to endure everything around the run as much as the run itself. That's what made this different to any race I'd done before. And though I had to beat myself up over my training regimes, I realised I had found myself doing some seriously mentally challenging training runs, many of which I had probably subconsciously tried to forget over the last couple of years. And, perhaps, the grilling I regularly gave myself was quite unnecessary. The mental and physical training I had done had already stood me in good stead.

Chapter Nineteen

The pressing questions

Four days till race day. This was our third day of trekking up the Everest trail and our eleventh day of trekking in all. It was the first day of our introduction to the giant grey boulders we would grow accustomed to the nearer to Everest we creeped. I had experienced a couple of really good days so far, managing the climbs in much more of a steady, ground-covering rhythm than I had at the start of the trek. Today, however, I felt bunged up with a second bout of the cold and was struggling for breath. We stopped at the halfway point we had agreed to meet at and I found my patience and generally cheery demeanour slipping away. I could feel a bad mood creeping up on me for which I couldn't quite pinpoint a reason. What was interesting was the fact that most of my fellow trekkers were also feeling the same. Perhaps it was the altitude or maybe too many days of our bodies feeling weary. Either way, our sombre mood seemed fitting as the next climb from here would take us up to the memorial site for fallen climbers, not just on Everest but surrounding mountains, too.

Thousands of climbers have died trying to scale and return from their beloved peaks. As a non-climber, it's difficult to get my head round. The list of hazards in the world of climbing, certainly on some of the highest peaks in the world, is long enough to make you believe the ceiling of the world is not meant for us. From organ failure, to exposure, to downright accidents, you are often battling dangers you can do little about.

But as a sportswoman I can empathise. When your sport is something that has consumed your life or perhaps given you life when you thought hope was lost, when your drive to succeed and reach this physical peak overtakes your desire to keep your body safe, it's difficult to argue with. There will always be a way around anything standing in your way. Even common sense or self-preservation.

There have been 292 recorded or suspected deaths on Everest alone. There hasn't been a death-free year since 1977. And in a world (certainly in my home country anyway) where accident and injury and danger are being minimised every day, it's very strange to look at the figures relating to the deaths on Everest and see that the numbers have increased over the past few years compared to 40 years ago.

This correlates, of course, with the commercialisation of Everest, whereby adventure companies now take groups upon groups of wealthy clients to the summit, meaning the number of people on Everest each year is significantly higher now than 40 years ago.

We entered the memorial ground on the hilltop, passing underneath strings of prayer flags overhead. Dozens of stupas stretched the length and breadth of the hilltop with more prayer flags strung between them. Each stupa had a plaque dedicated to a climber or team of climbers who had died on a mountain here in the Himalayas. There was the odd one dedicated to someone who had died elsewhere in the world and their climbing background meant a memorial on the Everest trail was deemed appropriate.

We took our time reading each name. I wondered if it had been worth it to them. Had they done everything they had wanted to do? Were they ready for the mountains to claim their bodies? A lot of these people, even if their bodies were found, would not be laid to rest. On Everest, certainly, it's usually not possible to bring anyone back and so these frozen bodies lie in plain sight all the way up the climbing route.

At the memorial ground, the memorial for Scott Fischer is among those here, too. Fischer was one of the leaders and owners of Adventure Consultants and was killed during the 1996 disaster on Everest. The disaster would form the basis for many films, including the questionable 2015 blockbuster *Everest*. Jon Krakauer, survivor of the 1996 disaster the film portrayed, and author of the book *Into Thin Air* which documents the disaster, described the film as 'total bull' with scenes describing events which didn't even happen.

Fischer's body also still lies, completely exposed and on display, on the fatal mountain, like many, many others. Horrendously, Fischer's corpse has become something of a tourist attraction in itself with climbers taking 'selfies' next to it. This is something I find hugely disrespectful to Fischer's family and the families of those who died alongside him.

Our group had become quite quiet and reflective as each memorial made us question ourselves and our own motives for being here. One plaque was dedicated to Hristo Prodanov, a Bulgarian mountaineer who had previously climbed Lhotse, the mountain next to Everest, without the use of supplementary oxygen. He had years and years of mountaineering experience behind him and had decided to attempt to summit Everest via the difficult west face, also without the use of supplementary oxygen. He did so alone and, though succeeding in summitting, was killed in a storm during the descent. Twenty years later his niece, Mariana Prodanov Maslarova, would attempt the same feat only to die from exposure at 8,700 metres, just 142 metres from the summit. Her plaque is on the opposite side of the same stupa on which her uncle's name is inscribed.

They'd each had a goal, just like most of us. The difference was that they'd decided they would risk death over a life without this accomplishment. Perhaps this wasn't how they had viewed it when planning and strategising, organising equipment and plotting how best to avoid accidents, exposure, sickness and the multitude of other life-threatening scenarios. But it's how I saw it as I stared at Maslarova's name on that plaque, her life now an etching on a piece of metal because she had wanted to finish what her uncle could not.

I had tears in my eyes by the time I read the last plaque that afternoon. My tears were for the waste of so much life and so much potential, more than anything. Not every climber remembered here could have been prepared for the end. They would have known the dangers, but a lot wouldn't have really expected it to happen to them. They would have had families and plans and things they wanted to do and see. Everest, or another mountain, had taken that from them. For others, I guessed maybe Everest, in those final hours, had given them everything they had yearned for in life. I thought about this as I listened to helicopters passing back and forth overhead, taking people to see the body-littered mountain. It was ironic and sad, and gives you a strange perspective on human nature.

Each of us left the memorial site taking a mental step back and looking at our own lives. This race, this whole experience, was something I had been fixated on reaching for two years. At what point did that fixation stop? At what point would I pull back and say, 'no'? I'd already forgone my health on more than one occasion. Perhaps it was time to realise some things are more important. Family and home was certainly foremost in my mind at that moment.

By the time we reached Lobuche, our last campsite on the trek, everyone was in a strange mood. It felt like a combination of weariness, reflection and tetchiness, and it would be fair to say each of us was ready for the end of the forthcoming race where there would be a bed, a shower and significantly fewer rocks.

24 November

A Message Home:

Writing this with no wifi at the moment just so it's ready to send if I get a glimmer of signal! Today (Friday) was tough for everyone I think. It seemed to go on for bloody ever, even though it was really only half a day's trek. We had slept at our highest camp yet which I think contributed to the general mood, and it was still -10°C at 6am. We had a climb of 700 metres to get to where we are now and it was probably the first day my mood has got darker and darker as I went along. This was eased slightly by the fact almost everybody is feeling the same today for some reason. It was not helped, however, by the sight of our campsite which is set on big stones and rough ground for the next two nights! The poor Sherpas had their work cut out getting the tents set up. Since Pherishe, the land has been boulderous and fairly bleak in comparison to the rest of the trek, but that can only mean we're close now! I'm not climbing Kala Patthar tomorrow, but I am considering going to the foot of the Khumbu Icefall where the current Everest Base Camp is. It's supposed to be an easy walk with only 400 metres of climbing. I really just want to get stuck into race day now!

The 'easy walk' to the current Everest Base Camp on the 25th was anything but. Most of us had tired bodies and still felt a little grumbly from the trek here. The inclines and declines and constant boulder-strewn terrain was all quite tiring to say the least. I spent most of the trek chastising myself for agreeing to go, as I had previously been determined to keep my legs as fresh as possible for the marathon. I had thought this was the easier option but I could feel my leg muscles searing with almost every step. What was I doing?! It wasn't until we had crossed to the middle of the glacier at the foot of the Khumbu Icefall that I stopped and thought, 'Ah, *this* is why I'm doing this!'

Base Camp is, essentially, a pile of rocks atop a lot of ice. Strewn around one particular pile of rocks is the memorabilia left by the many climbers and trekkers to pass through: scarves, t-shirts, photographs, signs, etc. These rocks seem to be level enough to pitch quite a few tents across. I'm still not entirely certain how the climbers (or more probably Sherpas) pitch a tent on top of these rocks, boulders and ice! Given my one and only solo tent pitching debacle, it's a knowledge field which is quite possibly always going to be beyond my understanding.

Everest is obscured from view at Base Camp but you can see the Khumbu Icefall where the climbers begin their ascent. At the time of the Swiss and British expeditions in 1952 and 1953, Base Camp was at Gorak Shep, where our start line would be. This meant each climber would be waking up on the first day of tackling Everest, knowing they still had at least two hours of trekking before the climbing even began. And given the fact that each climber should have spent two weeks trekking and acclimatising as we had just done, I imagine this thought was not a welcome one when all you wanted to do was get climbing!

A glacier shift many years ago changed the landscape in such a way that it became possible to pitch tents a lot closer to Everest, and so get the climbers climbing much sooner.

Having spent much of the trek marvelling at how the mountains felt close enough to touch, it was now actually possible, had we the inclination, to run over and feel the exposed gravel and rock of these beautiful monsters we had been creeping closer to. These freshly exposed mountainsides had been created by recent earthquakes.

The darker rocky face of the mountain had been stripped back to a light grey shale from a line around two-thirds of the way up. I imagined the glacier valley we had travelled up would have looked a lot different 60 years ago. We could now look straight back down the valley from the point we stood at, at the foot of the Khumbu Icefall. Tons of rocks and gravel looked to be freshly fallen (in the last few decades, anyway, which is 'freshly fallen' for geology geeks, right?) with hefty slabs and boulders of ice lying underneath. I wondered what Hillary and Tenzing had taken in before they tackled the nigh-on impossible feat in front of them.

For many climbers, this would be the last piece of 'real' ground they would feel, with rocks and earth still in sight, before entering a world of snow, ice, exposure and surreality.

This spot we stood on probably brought more relief to climbers than the summit of Everest itself. If they were seeing this spot, and this view, for a second time it meant they had survived Mount Everest. I imagine this brings a colossal sense of relief, gratitude and elation, and a new perspective on your own life.

We spent a good amount of time at Base Camp, taking many pictures alongside a few other trekkers and generally taking in the fact we were now standing almost on Everest, where some of the most famous, courageous, crazy mountaineers had also stood. Of course, there were no climbers here today, the climbing season for Everest being April and May.

As we made our way back to Lobuche, I realised that I really didn't mind the fact that my legs might be more tired tomorrow. If I had come all the way out to Gorak Shep and not trekked the extra distance to see and feel Base Camp, I would have kicked myself. The pictures alone made it worth it.

Chapter Twenty

The jinx that should never have been

26 November

It had arrived! The day before the race. The day I had quite literally dreamed of, usually waking up in a panic because I'd forgotten my entire race kit in the dream. But more than this, the day before the race had arrived and I felt amazing! While fellow trekkers had come down with traveller's diarrhoea for days at a time, my constitution had remained as sturdy as ever. While the altitude had given others crushing headaches, mine had been slight and passing.

While some had pulled out of the race altogether due to severe altitude sickness, I'd been fortunate enough to acclimatise fully. My heart rate was down and my oxygen was up, and at the height of Lobuche this was seriously impressing me! I felt like the luckiest girl alive at that moment.

I had lain in my tent the night before, heartened by the day's trek to Base Camp and fully accepting of the cold now. I thought to myself, I'm going to manage this race! I'm actually going to manage it! It was enough to bring tears to my eyes. I began to tentatively plan out the route and times to each checkpoint in my head. Based on the two training runs I had done up here, I had realised I could be quick. Not record-breakingly so, but not shabby either! We had been advised to double our normal marathon time for a realistic Everest race time. This had me around the eight-hour mark. However, if everything went to plan, I really felt I could complete this race in seven hours. I almost hushed myself at this thought. I didn't want to jinx it!

We were put through our final medical checks on 26 November. I had watched clips of these on YouTube from the 1999 race, and now I was queueing with the rest of the race participants waiting for my turn! It was madness. For me, it was like being a massive Star Wars geek then suddenly finding yourself on the Millennium Falcon, expected to fly the damn thing the next morning.

As we queued, we watched our tents being dismantled and packed on to the yaks for the last time. It was a grounding moment. We wouldn't camp together again! All that distance we had trekked, certainly up the Khumbu Valley to Everest, anyway, we would run tomorrow. We wouldn't see our yaks again until we had finished the race. I had washed my race kit the previous afternoon (since I had worn most of it during the trek) and was attempting to dry it outside my tent. Unfortunately, my socks were now solid, frozen batons and my T-shirt a similarly frozen slab. I had been trying in vain to defrost them while queueing.

Despite my not-yet-thawed kit, I was given the go-ahead to race the next day and bounced out of the lodge with the biggest smile I'd had during this whole trek. We crossed the leg-breaking, ankle-spraining ups and downs that would form the first three miles of our race, and I chirped away to my fellow participants, singing the only three lines of the song 'The Bonnie Banks o' Loch Lomond' I knew, over and over, most likely doing everyone's heads in. I grew more and more excited for the race ahead of us. I was surrounded by friends, in the middle of the Himalayas, on the eve of the biggest day of my life so far. It didn't get better than this.

We arrived at Gorak Shep and our lodge for the night. It was positioned on the edge of the lake, where our start would be, tomorrow morning at 6.30am. We had lunch, organised our things and tried to stay as warm as we could. At this height, the daytime heat we had felt earlier on the trek was no longer quite so apparent! Thankfully, my room for the night was upstairs, where the windows had a chance to just about defrost during the day, so weren't coated in two inches of ice as they were downstairs.

Walking into the lodge you'd be forgiven for thinking you had a sudden bout of altitude sickness as the floor sloped this way and that, and sent you swaying slightly as you walked in. It was also fairly dark with only a few windows letting in some light. As much as we could, we stayed outside where it seemed more welcoming.

We were expected on the start line that afternoon at three o'clock for a briefing, though photos were really the main reason for this, I'm sure! As I waited for 3pm to roll around, I wondered why I was beginning to feel a bit queasy. Perhaps, despite being well acclimatised before, I wasn't dealing well with the height now. Or perhaps our lunch had been a little grease-heavy, consisting of fried Spam, fried Tibetan bread and coleslaw.

I headed out for the briefing, determined to ignore whatever this queasiness was. We stood for a good many photos and I felt my chirpy mood sliding away as the queasiness turned into something a bit more nagging. Someone told me I didn't look so good and that the colour was starting to drain from my face. With two other runners standing in front of me, I tried to make myself sick. Maybe I just needed to throw up and I'd be fine. It didn't help, however.

Beginning to feel shaky, I made my way to my room. The stairs were even more exhausting than they had been a few hours ago. Gods, what was wrong with me? After an hour or so of lying restlessly in my sleeping bag, I suddenly had to rush to the 'bathroom' at the end of the first floor hall. The lodge had a hill at the back of it which our floor seemed to run level with, meaning the toilet we had could, once again, be a hole in the floor. I threw up for several seconds into this hole in the ground. I was throwing up hard enough to not be able to breathe. When it stopped and I could get a panicked breath in it was only a few seconds before I started throwing up again. And then again. Someone heard me and shouted to see if I was okay. I answered a shaky, 'Yeah.' I'd be damned if a bit of sickness was going to ruin this race for me now. I threw up again, stomach contracted tightly in on itself, making me gasp and splutter. Someone else asked through the door if I needed a doctor. After a few seconds of silence, I finally whimpered, 'Maybe.' However, there was very little the doctor could do. She gave me an anti-sickness tablet and some salts, and offered a shoulder to cry on.

I just wanted my mum. I told the doctor this as I quite literally cried all over her shoulder. Thank God for our group doctor. She did her very best to comfort me before leaving me to get some rest.

The anti-sickness tablet came straight back up minutes later and this was to be followed by an entire night of stumbling in the sub-zero darkness to and from the hole in the ground at the end of the corridor. The diarrhoea started early on in the evening and continued until the morning, long after the sickness had become a horrible dry retching because there was nothing left to bring up. I had never felt as far from home as I did that night. The strength with which I wanted to be back with my family around me was overwhelming and made me realise, in one of the harshest ways possible, that all that really mattered in my life was family and home.

In between going back and forth to the hole in the ground, I lay in my sleeping bag, shaking violently from the combined effects of the cold and shock of whatever sickness this was. To begin with I cried. I had come this far; two years of training my heart out through injuries, tears and more tears. I'd been supported by so many people who believed in me, and now that the time was here, I was going to let them all down. I was going to let down the charity and all the ex-soldiers I was raising money for. And, on top of this, I was going to let myself down.

But I had a lot of hours of lying in that sleeping bag. The tears grew exhausting after a while, and I grew angry. So much for all the 'meant to be' shit. Was this 'meant to be'? What sort of cruel shit is that? Everything falls into place right up until fucking D-Day then it gets swiped away!

I wasn't having it. Absolutely fucking not. I had not worked my arse off for two years then spent two weeks freezing it off, dragging myself out to the middle of nowhere to not do this thing. Yes, I was exhausted just getting to the end of the corridor to throw my guts up. Yes, my head spun and I started breathing hard as soon as I raised myself from my sleeping bag. But if I could still stand in the morning I would be on that fucking start line. There was no question.

Chapter Twenty-One

Race day

5.30am, 27 November

There was a rapping on my door and heavy footsteps up and down the corridor outside my room. Race day had arrived. The Sherpas were waking the Everest Marathon race participants, and everyone was rousing. Last pieces of race kit were being packed and sleeping bags and main bags were being loaded, ready to be taken back down to Namche for us.

I pushed my feet into my hiking boots, as I had been doing all night, feeling as pale and drawn as I probably looked, and stood up with a slight sway. I made my way to the end of the corridor with my toothbrush in hand, stopping at the end to lean my whole body against the wall and catch my breath.

My legs wanted me to sit down; my spinning head wanted me to sit down. But my unquellable stomach told me nothing was going to bring me comfort this morning so there was no point. It was -17°C, I had no energy and I was now out of my insulated sleeping bag. Hypothermia was not beyond the bounds of possibility. I had spent the night in my trekking trousers and two fleeces in order to go back and forth to the toilet without having to re-dress every time. The cuffs of my outer fleece were now crisp with frozen sick.

At this point I wasn't even thinking of the race. I had the mammoth task of getting all my things into two bags and myself dressed in something that wasn't now covered in sick. And right now I didn't even have the energy to go to the toilet and brush my teeth.

The person currently using the toilet left just in time as my bowels decided once again to evacuate all contents, despite the fact that there was nothing left to evacuate. We'd been doing this all night, for Christ's sake!

'Give me a break,' I muttered to myself, managing just in time to drag my trousers down and squat over the hole in the ground for what felt like the 453rd time. I knew there were people waiting outside and in any other circumstance the noises coming from this toilet would have caused me much embarrassment. But I was too exhausted to feel embarrassment; too exhausted to even muster mild acknowledgement this morning. Unless it was someone offering me a time machine, a miracle pill or a flight back home, I didn't have the patience or energy to care.

After breaking the ice on the water barrel to wash away the mess, I traipsed back down the corridor to start the process of shoving things in a bag and hoping the thing zipped shut when I was done. It was dark and we didn't have the luxury of lights so everything was to be done by head torch.

This wasn't how I had envisaged the morning of the biggest race of my life. In my ideal world, I would have had my race bag packed the night before, ready for every eventuality yet still exceptionally light. I would have taped my shins, knees and ankles before bed and spent a restful night with compression socks over the tape. My three numbers would all be fixed in place and ready to go. All I'd have to do in the morning would be to put my sleeping bag in its case and hand everything to our head Sherpa before I went downstairs for a hearty breakfast of sweet porridge.

Instead, the floor was littered with every item imaginable from where I'd tipped bags out to find hydration tablets, Imodium, batteries, my head torch, toothbrush and toothpaste, with no thought for the effort it would take to fix in the morning. I had been trying not to projectile vomit at the time. Such things hadn't been occurring to me.

My current state of mind and the fact that light was limited was not conducive to pinning race numbers on or taping up muscles, either. If I hadn't used up all my tears last night I would have cried at the prospect. By the time this was done and my sleeping bag was packed away I was breathing heavily again and trying to quell the sick feeling in my stomach.

Our poor Head Sherpa came bustling in, clearly stressed to find my main bag only half packed.

'Very sorry to hear about your illness,' he said with a slightly manic cheerfulness as he grabbed random items and started throwing them into my main bag, some of which I would need for the race. It was like a comedy sketch, him throwing items into the big purple bag and me taking them straight back out again behind him.

Eventually, and by some miracle, I found myself down in the dimly lit dining room 15 or so minutes before we were due outside. Most race participants were trying to get some breakfast into themselves, the overall mood sombre. At best it had been a bitterly cold night for most, with minimal sleep from the thumping back and forth along the corridor outside their rooms by either me or the other few people who had also got sick.

I knew without even thinking about it that I couldn't stomach any kind of breakfast. I had been given a bottle of Coke which I was letting go flat. Considering the race like a prisoner waiting to go to the gallows (yes, a tad dramatic now I come to think of it!), I knew I had no source of energy in my body. Any food that had been in my system now wasn't, one way or another, and at this altitude we were all burning calories at rest, never mind throughout a night of retching and shaking.

I barely spoke to anyone except to refuse food and resorted to the only preparation I knew I could do, which was to try to instil some determination in myself. Even just to start this race. All I had to do was get to checkpoint one; that was only three miles. Even on my worst days of training I could manage three miles.

I didn't tell myself I could pull out at checkpoint one. I don't really know that I promised myself anything if I reached that point. It was just a case of 'all you have to do is get to checkpoint one'. Maybe I thought the time it took to get there would give the running hormones in my body a chance to kick in and I'd miraculously find a reserve of energy.

With a dusky light beginning to creep across the pale lake bed that would be our start line, 50 runners traipsed outside. Only 40 of us would finish. Down jackets, gloves and hats were being hugged tightly as most of us watched the Nepalese runners bouncing around in front of us in their shorts and T-shirts, apparently oblivious to the fact that it was -17°C and us foreign runners were likely to lose our kneecaps to frostbite if we dressed as they did! I stood in one spot, shifting my feet around for the ten minutes or so we had to wait. My bottle of flat Coke was in one hand, my bottle of water in the other, and both were tucked under my armpits. I don't remember saying much to anyone around me apart from the odd 'Good luck.' 'This is it,' I murmured to myself as our guide shouted for us to take off our down jackets with two minutes to go. We reluctantly dumped them on a sheet of tarpaulin lying just off to the side, and no amount of hugging yourself could stop the sub-zero temperature pouncing on your skin. I had on base layers and sports-tech overlayers but I may as well have been naked.

With 90 seconds to go my hands started to grow painful. Now, I'm from Scotland and I do a lot of outdoor work. I have had painfully cold hands before: cold enough to make you cry. But that was nothing compared to how painful my hands were going to get during the first three miles of this race. I'm talking 'someone has taken a hammer to them and broken every bone' kind of painful.

I would like to say that the countdown began and I readied myself for the race of my life. I'd like to say 'Go!' was shouted and I heroically set off at a good, strong pace, starting as I meant to go on. I didn't.

As time was counted down, I stood, stony faced and cursing every stupid idea that had brought me to this godforsaken place. As 'Go' was shouted, I set off at a walk towards the hill out of the frozen lake that would take us to the first hell-like glacier of this race. The first few hundred metres were sand and, though the Nepalese runners flew over it like jackrabbits on speed, I knew

I'd keel over and likely need airlifting to hospital after 15 seconds if I even tried to jog.

The climb started and even at a walk I had my hands on my thighs, leg muscles feeling like they hadn't been exercised in three years. We had trekked over this section three times and this would be the fourth crossing so we already knew that the perilous descents and steep climbs over the glacier field seemed never ending because it all looked the same. You couldn't let your attention waver from the grey rocks and ice or you would almost certainly break some part of your body.

There were two layers of thin fabric between my legs and the frigid air around me. Even at my most energetic I think the muscular response in my limbs would have been limited. But now I couldn't get them to react to the ground as I was seeing it. I needed to get down these slopes quickly so I wasn't lagging behind too badly on the steep climbs. To have the sweep team at my heels this early on would surely only end in my failure before the race had really begun. But if I let gravity do its thing my legs wouldn't move quickly enough to keep up, let alone lift over and around every rock in time. My gait turned into a stilted, pantomime-like jog.

The gloves on my hands may as well have been chucked in the bin back at Base Camp. They were utterly useless. The two bottles of liquid in my hands were essentially two blocks of ice against my skin, and it felt like the bones were shattering inside my fingers. My lungs wouldn't fill with air properly because it was too cold, and no amount of breathing through a buff was warming it. I got to the top of one climb, around a mile in, legs feeling as if I was pulling them through mud and my whole body screaming because it had nowhere near enough energy or oxygen to perform properly. I crouched, curling myself as tightly together as possible, and tried to breathe, which turned into something of a pained moan. My two bottles were under my armpits as I tried to clench and unclench my hands in an unsuccessful attempt to push blood into them.

'Get your chest up!' A runner from my group was coming up the climb behind me. 'You don't have to move, just get your chest up,' he said to me kindly but with enough urgency to be serious. You wouldn't think these words would have much effect, seeing them on paper, but at the time they were the only things I had to cut through the environment around me that seemed to be crushing the life out of me. They were compassion, kindness and a genuine concern for my well-being. At this point I was a weedy kid out of school squaring up to Mike Tyson and having every blow I attempted hit back at me with ten times the power. These words were all I had, right now, to dodge those blows.

It reminded me of the camaraderie and team spirit we had developed over the last two weeks among our groups. We had all been through some rough patches during the two weeks it had taken to get here, and we had bared all to one another. And now, when I was at the point of feeling physically crushed and defeated, this fellow runner was here with the words and support I needed. At the very least it would help keep me alive. I straightened, though every part of my body wanted me to stay crouched on that spot. I nodded to my friend, unable to speak but he could see I would heed his advice. We would at least reach checkpoint one.

The sight of the green lodge roof in Lobuche, appearing from around a corner, was one of the most relieving sights I had ever seen. I can't explain why; it was a checkpoint with a table and some warm, weak juice. There was no fire to warm yourself by, no bed to rest in, no helicopter in which to fly home (God, that would have been good!). But I had told myself I just had to get to checkpoint one and now I was a few metres away. I felt a basic reward response, I suppose.

I reached the marshal who had been our group leader during the trek, and the sight of her smiling face was as big a comfort as I could have asked for at that time. Aside from a helicopter, of course. Word had reached her of my sickness and the hug she gave me helped build a tiny bit of determination to get to checkpoint two.

'The sun will be up soon,' she told me encouragingly. 'That was the coldest section and it's over now.'

I nodded, still not doing well with the speaking.

She gave me her mittens to use instead of my gloves and told me to swing my arms in circles to try to get the blood back into them. I genuinely would not have been surprised to find black patches on my hands when I took those gloves off. Luckily all skin was un-frostbitten. I binned my bottle of Coke, untouched, as it was completely frozen and would only keep me cold if I held on to it.

It's easy sometimes to look back on tough races and think 'it really wasn't that bad', forgetting most of the details and feelings from that time. However, I don't think there will ever be a point in my life when I look back on the first three miles of the Everest Marathon and forget how bad they really were. It will always be in the back of my mind as the worst three miles I have ever endured.

When I look back, the only thing that kept me moving over that section was the hard fact that *there was no other way*. Even if I had pulled out of the race, I would have had to cross that glacier section on foot. I literally had no choice.

The sun did indeed rise, halfway between checkpoints one and two, and though I was not immediately warmed, the difference felt miraculous.

My progress to checkpoints two and three was spurred on by smiling marshals who had become my friends during the trek and who had words of kindness and encouragement. Friendly trekkers also helped to push me onwards. One extravagant Italian gentleman kissed my hand and told me I was doing fantastically. In any other circumstance this would have been less than desired but as it stood I could have married him there and then. From mile four to nine would turn out to be the best section of my race. Perhaps I had been right: I *had* found a reserve of running energy after checkpoint one. I didn't feel full of energy by any means but I was able to keep up a rhythm and cover the rocky ground sometimes among, sometimes in front of, other runners.

But this reserve of energy was not three days of carb loading, it wasn't two days of rest, it wasn't a restful night's sleep and it wasn't a hearty breakfast. It was short-lived.

After checkpoint three, we had a few climbs and descents during which I focussed on simply getting up and getting down. I was finding I was coming across sections I didn't recognise since it had been such a long trek with a lot of similar rocks. So, as one section I didn't recognise stretched on and on, I puttered out. I don't know how else to describe it. I didn't think to myself 'I'll just stop now', my legs did it completely of their own accord. I bent over, hands on thighs, and cried. It wasn't many tears, more like dry crying really, but what was strange was the fact that it wasn't an emotional response. I'd shuttered off the magnitude of the task in my head and had been refusing to let myself feel it. These tears were purely a physical response to the stress I was starting to force my body through.

'Fuck,' I said to myself. 'How am I supposed to get through an entire fucking marathon?'

It was the first time I had properly considered the logistics of this thing since last night, when I had mentally steeled myself to be on the start line this morning.

It was at this point that the group of guys I had been just a little in front of passed by. Always with a smile on each of their faces – though I knew they too had found some parts challenging so far – they gave me some words of encouragement on their way past as I tried to walk off my bout of exhaustion. For the next three or four minutes I picked up to a jog which would soon drop away to a walk. I'd pick it up again and it would drop away just as fast.

'Shit,' I was starting to panic now. Hands on hips, I shook my head. My body wasn't going to get me through this. 'Shit, shit, shit.'

Up ahead, one guy from the group that had just passed seemed to be emerging from the side of the track, presumably from answering the call of nature. Sam spotted me quite clearly lagging. What I didn't realise at that point was that this man would end up staying with me throughout the rest of the race, despite the fact he could complete it considerably faster than I was ever going to manage. Sam had run races all over the world, including a hundred-mile ultra, and was obviously not lacking in competitive spirit (none of us were). And yet he was willing to give up knowing how fast he could really complete the world-renowned Everest Marathon, and any chance at a decent placing, just to make sure I got through it. This will be enough to maintain my faith in humanity for a good many years, especially since some of the episodes he would have to put up with in the coming hours should have earned him a separate medal altogether.

'The next checkpoint isn't far now,' he lied, very convincingly, as I approached where he was waiting for me on the track.

'Really?' With the lack of any familiar features around me and a landscape that didn't seem to be changing, I was losing the mental drive to keep going. At this stage, I was willing to grasp at anything that might convince my mind to keep telling my legs to continue moving. Even if it was just the idea of another checkpoint being close.

'I reckon we're over 17km now. That's less than 2km to go to the checkpoint.' His maths might have been correct, but it didn't feel like 'less than 2km'. The repetitiveness of my surroundings was, thankfully, broken up by having some company with me now, and together we trundled along at a steady pace.

Over the next few miles, I forced myself into a routine of running or jogging the flats and downhills and one-foot-in-front-of-the-other walking the uphills. Even if they were only a slight incline, I treated them as an uphill, since a slight incline still felt like a leg-buster. My mind could deal with this routine, and only a couple of times over the next few miles did I have to stop quite inexplicably and let my body gather itself.

But there were two big climbs to come. The height gained by reaching the top of each would be almost equalled by the height lost on the other side of them but that was little comfort to me on this side. Down at Namche, at a mere 3,200m, climbing one short flight of stairs had been enough to make me breathless and a little light-headed. Our trek up the valley to Base Camp had been full of rocky climbs where we would have to stop every hundred steps or so to breathe through our arses. And that had been fully fuelled, without 16 miles of exertion behind us.

By the time we reached the start of the first big climb to the spectacular Tengboche Monastery, I had begun to recognise my surroundings again. This only meant I had a good half hour or so to dwell on the impending doom approaching. I may be wrong, but I'm fairly certain only the Nepalese runners would have run this climb. Even at sea level it would have been a bit stiff, but at this height, one's legs were screaming within 20 seconds. I stopped frequently – sometimes to double over and try to breathe, sometimes to cry.

I had been wondering how I was going to get to the finish line for a good few miles now, and the hopelessness of the situation and the helplessness of my body were definitely beginning to bring about an emotional response, not just physical exhaustion.

We finally crested the hill, emerging at Tengboche Monastery and our fifth checkpoint. To see our Sherpa guide Neema and travel writer Kelly at the station was a welcome relief. Neema had been such a calming, strong figure throughout the trek, always there to help. Even now he was quietly but determinedly making certain my running buddy ate the bowl of porridge he had put in his hands. I must have still looked queasy enough that Neema could see I really wasn't going to manage any.

I remember this being the point, despite the smiling, welcoming faces of Kelly and Neema, at which I began to get angry again. Angry at my body for failing me at the most crucial point, and angry at whatever forces were at play to make this happen. I had to blame something, so invisible forces would have to do. I was also feeling distinctly guilty for holding my very kind running buddy back, though he had refused to carry on without me each time I told him to.

I stopped to rest for a far shorter period of time than I should have before setting off over the other side of the hill with a strong sense of stubbornness instilled in my brain. I would force my damned body through this race whether it liked it or not. The strongest version of me would have kicked my arse seeing me crying as I had been. How dare I let myself be so weak. How dare my trained body not perform. Sure, I hadn't trained as an elite athlete but I sure as hell had trained it to be resilient. So what was this? I wasn't having it. I deliberately set off as my running partner was still trying to finish the very full bowl of Neema's porridge. Bless him.

The descent was the steepest on the course and there were two options. You could either bullet straight down the side, presumably taking the shortcuts the locals and porters used, or you could take the trekkers' path that zig-zagged down. Even the zig-zagging path was rough enough and steep enough to pose a serious risk to one's ankles; the shortcut would have been suicidal to anyone who wasn't a local. I set off down the path at as fast a pace as I calculated was safe, ignoring the battering and jarring sensations up my legs and through my knees. It had always been my aim, during training for this marathon, to keep everything intact. I needed to be physically ready for the Everest Marathon. Everything needed to be in working order. I was here now, and there was nothing after this to be in one piece for. I could push everything to within an inch of breaking point, batter every joint, pound every fibre, and it wouldn't matter as long as I got to that finish line. I could hop over it if I had to. It would have been quite liberating if I hadn't been so intensely focussed on the ground and where I was putting my feet. I went over on each ankle twice but managed to stay upright. It only fuelled the stubborn, seething anger that was still pulsing in my mind.

The next climb wouldn't be long after I reached the bottom of this hill and I was ready for it. I would do this thing if it bloody well killed me. I was back down at the level of the river, crossing another suspension bridge and passing through a small gathering of homes and teahouses. I greeted trekkers and locals with a chirpy 'Namaste!' and forced a cheerful, capable demeanour on myself. I had this in hand. Fake it till you make it is the expression, I believe.

Just as I was leaving the settlement, Sam caught up with me, surprised at how much ground I had covered so quickly. Again, I told him to carry on without me, and again he told me not to be silly. We started the second climb together. It, too, zig-zagged but had far more boulders, plus rocky steps and slabs to climb and prayer stones on most corners. In my head I remembered this section as being long but in one piece – as in, once I'd reached the top, that would be it, done. It would be flat or downhill almost all the way to Namche. I was refusing to think about the last six-mile loop at this point. The thought of this being the last big effort powered me, along with the sense of stubbornness still lingering. We would storm up three or four turns then take a rest for a few seconds before continuing. And as we neared the top, I pushed my exhausted legs on. I could do this; it really wasn't much further.

Except that when we got to the top, we realised it wasn't really the top at all. There was another uphill section, and then another. And though these weren't steep climbs compared to the two previous ascents, they were still uphill and they went on and on. I felt like I was in a colder, harsher, more mountainous version of *Alice in Wonderland*, the difference being that there was no smiling cat, just rocks, yak dung and that feeling of hope being snatched away over and over.

'I fucking hate mountains,' I said, collapsing on a boulder after an hour or so. I bent over my knees once more, breathing hard. Helplessness was beginning to seep back in. 'I never want to see the godforsaken things again.' I truly meant it. At this point in time, the Himalayas were no longer magical and breathtaking. They were a never-ending cycle of rocks and hills with a backdrop of bigger rocks and bigger hills. There really was something to be said for the beaches of Hawaii.

My resolute stubbornness was shattered after the fifth or sixth crushing disappointment at finding yet another gradient to climb. It wasn't until a mind-numbing amount of time had passed, and I'd shed several more tears, that we finally reached the third to last checkpoint. It was situated at a lodge which, sadly, would burn down a couple of days later. This station was manned by a doctor we hadn't yet met, and we tried to look at least semi-human as we passed through. We weren't getting to this stage and being pulled off the course for appearing in need of resuscitation, that was for sure.

For the first time since the trek began, the sky had started to cloud over. The temperature difference was almost the same as when the sun slipped behind a mountain. The layers I had stripped off earlier in the race when the heat had started to build were quickly put back on as sweat started to go cold on my skin.

Thankfully, the climbing did stop and the course became undulating. I'm not sure how much more my mind could have taken had the hills continued. I had now spent seven hours forcing my body to perform under extreme stress, my mind to stay strong, picking it up and forcing it on every time I broke down physically and emotionally. I had drained every resource I had at my disposal. What I went into now was something in the realms of a numb, monotone existence. My mind stopped processing anything beyond the next step and the image of the finish line. My body stopped really feeling anything other than the same tedious all-over exhaustion that settled in every fibre. I ran. Not as fast as a machine, but as brain-dead as one. I ran until I couldn't. Then I stopped for a few seconds or minutes. Then I ran again. Over and over.

My poor running buddy was worried about me, I could tell. He would ask me to just stop and rest, take it easy. I'd shake my head.

'It'll only take longer.' I'm sure the look in my eye must have been pretty dead and glazed by this point.

And this was how we reached the second to last checkpoint, but not before passing a team of Gurkhas in the scrubby undergrowth by one of the paths. They didn't seem as impressed by our running antics as some of the trekkers we had met, funnily enough.

The checkpoint was at the start of the Thamo loop. This was a three-mile out-and-back from the village of Namche that would make up the last six miles of the marathon. This meant that this checkpoint was almost spitting distance from the finish line in the village. As we headed away from it and the friendly marshal, I refused to look back at the village. I refused to think about what was behind me, that the finish line was just there. It may as well have been on the other side of Everest for how near it felt in my head.

My deadened state only worsened as this section became much like the never-ending hill. The turnaround point was always 'just around the corner' and yet we would be met with another section, another part of the valley and no turnaround point. Because it was an out-and-back, we came across many other runners on their way back, all in varying states. Some had become sick on the course; some were just exhausted. It was going to be a battle to the end for most.

At one point I thought I could see the turnaround point. We passed through the prayer hut, just as we had on our training run, and swung to the left to run alongside a stone wall that split the path. A runner a quarter of a mile back had told us we were close now; that it wasn't far. He'd had a massive smile on his face and offered a big hug to match. This was it, praise the Lord, it was here.

Except that it wasn't. The runner had lied, and this area *exactly* matched the next valley. We had yet another section to cross. At that point of realisation, I stopped dead.

'Please, please tell me it's not over that hill,' I begged my friend, shaking my head as if he had a gun pointed at me or something.

He looked pained. 'I'm sorry.'

In full-on amateur-dramatic style I bent over and cried very, very loudly. It was a few minutes before I got my head through this last big disappointment, but once I did I let the resolute numbness take over again. We made our way, section by section, to the turnaround point where a ribbon was tied to each of our bags. We were on the home straight now.

In much the same *Alice in Wonderland* style the rest of the race had taken, the last three-mile stretch to

Namche Bazaar elongated to at least ten times its length. The last turn before the descent on to the cobbled streets of Namche involved passing around the side of a hill, over a helipad and through a stone archway. The cloud had now rolled in across the hills and it was difficult to tell how far we were from those points. As it started to look as if we might be approaching them, I pointed and tried to speak.

'Hill, round, helicopter.' I couldn't even form a sentence. Sam took a few seconds to answer.

'Yeah.'

It was a good enough answer for me.

Passing through the main street of Namche was a powerful experience. Runners who had already finished, the people who had become my friends over the last two weeks, were waiting on the street to cheer me on and keep me going. I rounded the last corner and up the steps to the finish line. As an aside, the cruelty of putting the finish line of the Everest Marathon at the top of a set of steps is quite unforgiveable! I had sent my running buddy on ahead to get a photo for my sponsors, and he and the rest of the crew were waiting to catch me as I all but collapsed in a crying heap once I was over the line. I cried with relief and exhaustion and from being so utterly overwhelmed at the support I had around me. I was so busy crying, in fact, that I forgot to accept my medal until one of the Sherpas came over to place it around my neck.

Holding the small gold medallion in my hands, I turned it over and read the word on the back through teary eyes. It simply said '2017'. Those four numbers inscribed on the back were probably the most meaningful I'd ever read.

I had done it. I'd completed the 2017 Everest Marathon.

Epilogue

End of a chapter

31 December 2017

It's the last day of the year and, as with every 31 December, I'm feeling wistful and nostalgic. It's silly, really, and perhaps only a characteristic of those with a tendency to write and dream and imagine on far too frequent a basis! This year has seen every emotion I thought it was possible to have: tears, pain, laughter, joy, confidence lows and confidence highs. It's been filled with lasting images of some of the most breathtaking sights, the feeling of wild weather against my skin and, most bizarrely, it's seen this crazy ambition I had thought was so many galaxies away come to fruition in a way I couldn't even have dreamed.

Two days after the marathon, we trekked back to Lukla from Namche Bazaar. It would be fair to say most of us were pining for home, a hot shower and jelly babies. We did the trek to the airport in one day rather than the two it had taken us on the way up, as we were largely descending. On tired legs, and still feeling ill from my bout of food poisoning, it did not feel like we were doing much descending. Every person in the group had lost drastic amounts of weight and so none of us had much energy for the chit-chat we'd been full of at the start of our adventure. At each rest point, we would mainly talk about what food we were going to have the second we touched down at home. I, for one, never wanted to see, smell or eat garlic ever again. Ever. Again. The detail to which each meal was planned gave some indication of just how many calories we had worn through during our time in the Himalayas.

The joys of a hot shower and comfortable bed were kept from us a little longer as we were grounded at Lukla airport due to cloudy conditions. Lack of communication, language barriers and money changing hands on the sly somewhere made the whole situation quite frustrating once the weather cleared and we still weren't on our plane. Luckily, our Sherpa guide managed to get us on a plane on the third day and with pure relief (our flight from Kathmandu back to London had been growing closer by the second) we touched down in the Nepalese capital. The sudden madness of traffic and bustle came as a shock to the system after the peace of the Himalayas, and we had to remind ourselves once more of how not to be run over.

With a day or so to wander the city before our departure, I found myself trying to pool my thoughts and feelings about the last two years. I was still processing the past month and the sudden turn of events, with the exhaustion and sickness still lingering. That period was coming to an end. The book was about to close and I wasn't sure how I felt about it all.

During the last few weeks of my training for Everest, I can honestly say I had started to grow sick of running. It had been a long two years of experiencing the success, joy and discovery of the run, but also two years of frustration, failure and exhaustion. Before I left for Nepal, I had vowed to quit endurance sport after Everest. And I had meant it, certainly consciously, anyway. I would take up 'normal' exercise, start to practise yoga, swim more regularly and devote time to looking after myself. I would no longer let endurance sport envelop my entire life.

It's been almost a month since I touched down in drizzly Edinburgh where I immediately located a toilet and spent a full 15 minutes enjoying everything from the doors to the taps to the toilet seat (it was amazing). I've eaten, slept, eaten and slept some more since returning, and all without a thought for training plans, kinesiology tape, ketogenic foodstuffs or how long my trainers might last. It's been great. But I'm starting to feel the first twinges of restlessness. I know, deep down, I won't be able to lead a 'normal' life. I won't be able to trundle down to the gym a couple of times a week to keep my waistline or blood pressure down (whichever one is more important these days). I won't be able to potter through the coming years, aiming at earning a little money to settle down and continue trundling. These aren't post-marathon blues; I don't feel frustrated or sad or emotional. In a way, I have the clearest outlook I've ever had.

Endurance sport has allowed me to set clear goals, with a structured training plan to reach each of these goals. That in itself gives a person self-discipline, self-respect and a sense of strength you never knew you had. The charity work has given me a purpose I believe in.

Curled up on the sofa with a blanket around my legs, watching the snow start to fall outside, and with Disney's *Tangled* on the TV, I can't stop thinking about it. If the past two years could give me this much, it could do the same for veterans. Especially those suffering from PTSD. The focus, the structure, the new-found self-respect – it's what these guys need.

There was an idea beginning to tease at the edge of my mind. Being among crazy-minded endurance athletes for an entire month had enlightened me about the extent of the mad-hat races out there. There were one or two in particular I thought might just be crazy enough to grab the attention of an even wider audience, creating a bigger platform for veteran recovery. The Run Watson Run campaign had raised over £2,500. But with a bigger project, aimed at corporate sponsorship rather than public, I estimated (from my comfy spot on the sofa) it would be possible to raise several times that over a further two years.

Of course, this was all hypothetical. I was due to start stretching on a mat and enjoying walks in the countryside next month. I wasn't about to start thinking about the ecstasy of crossing an ultramarathon finish line after hours of chemical and physical brilliance, or the tantalising fear of a long training run I wasn't sure I could manage, or the thrill of a harsh wind whipping over my skin atop an exposed mountain somewhere. These were things I *used* to do. Stories to tell the grandchildren.

All the same, maybe I'd just have a quick look at some of the adventures I'd heard of in the Amazon jungle, I thought to myself as I pulled the laptop over and clicked open Google ...